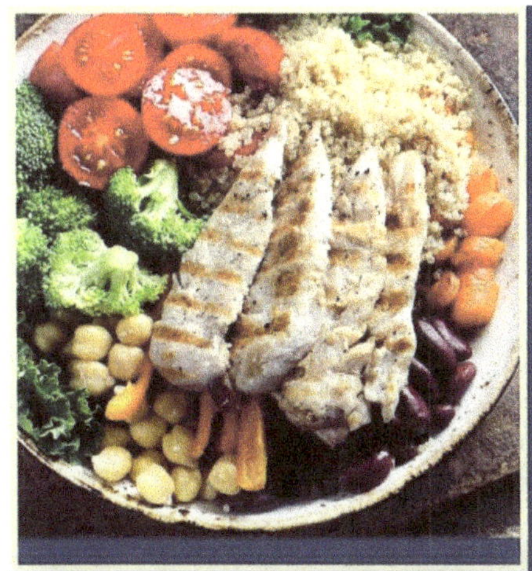

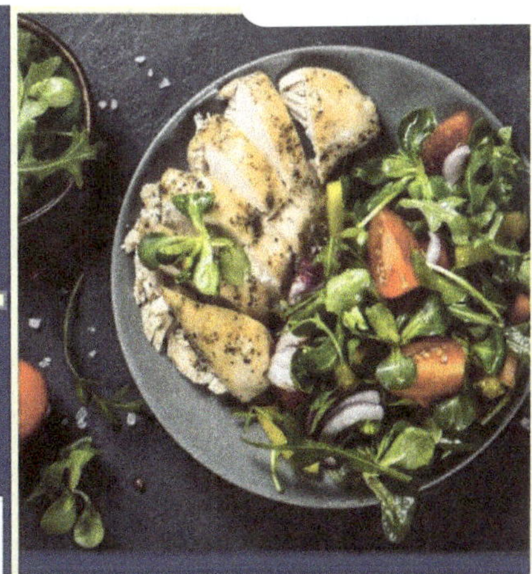

HEALTHY DAYS MEAL PLAN

LAURIE W. LAMB

THE COMPLETE & EASY

DIVERTICULITIS

Diet COOKBOOK

QUICK AND SIMPLE NUTRITIOUS RECIPES | MEAL PLAN INCLUDED.

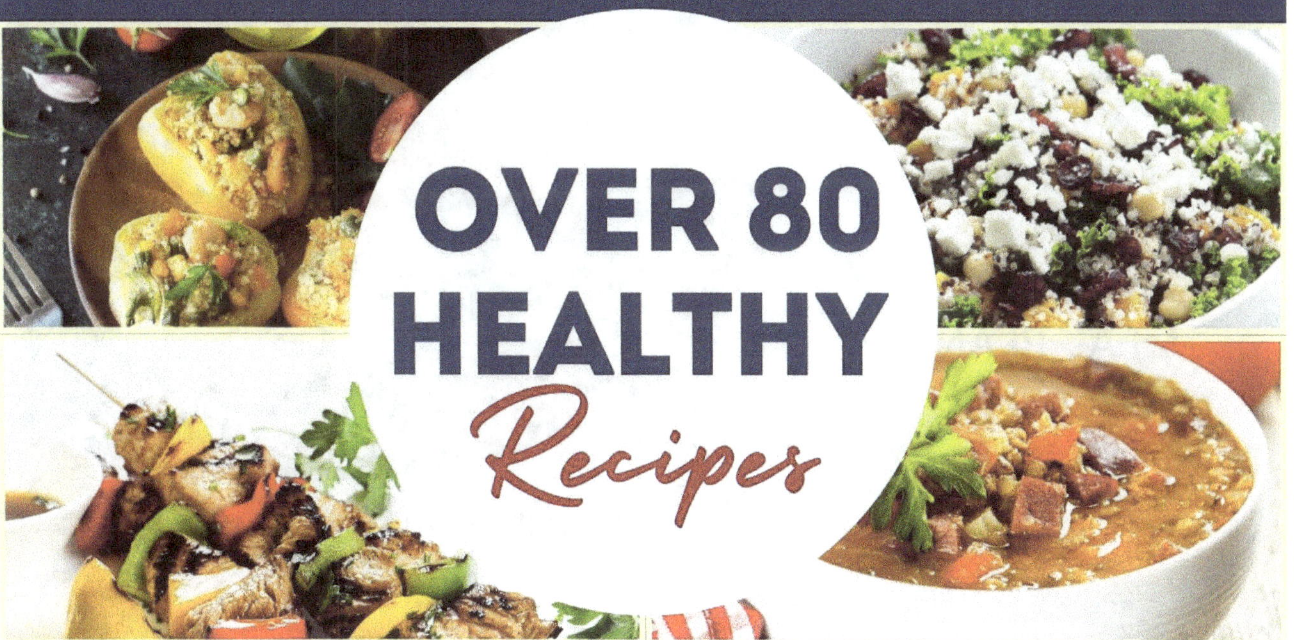

DIVERTICULITIS DIET

COOKBOOK

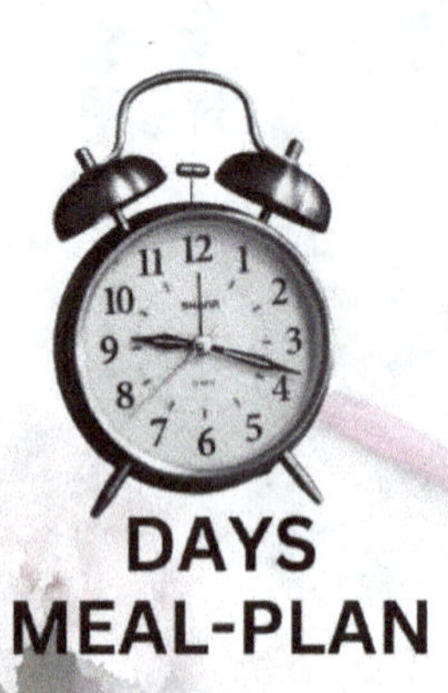

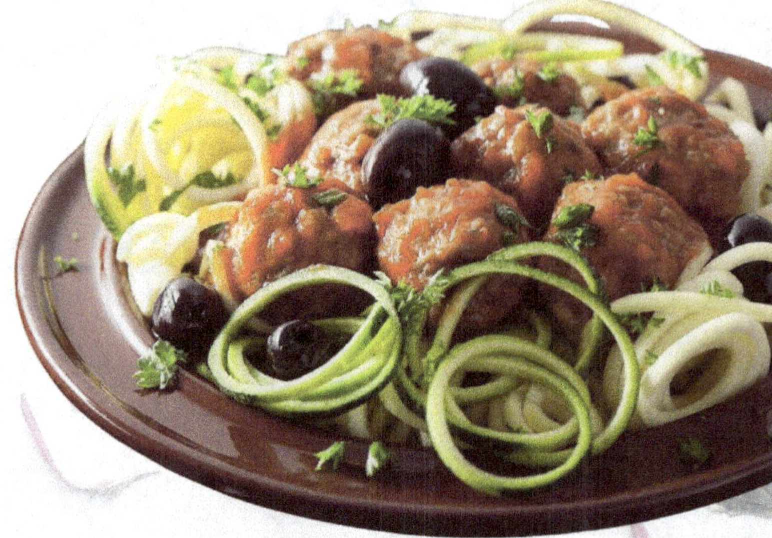

LAURIE W. LAMB

The complete & Easy
Diverticulitis Diet Cookbook

This cookbook is devoted to individuals who have valiantly navigated the complicated roads of the diverticulitis diet. Your path is one of strength and tenacity, punctuated by the daily balancing act of food and well-being. You confront the challenge of making every meal a healthier option, which demonstrates your steadfast attitude.

In the kitchen, you convert materials into nourishment, creating foods that satisfy not just your nutritional requirements but also your taste senses and heart. This book is an homage to your imagination, persistence, and tenacity. It is a tribute to the numerous hours spent studying, planning, and cooking meals that are both healing and satisfying.

May each dish in this compilation bring you comfort and joy. As you read through these pages, know that you are not alone on this journey. You are a member of a community that understands the challenges and accomplishments of living with diverticulitis. We honor your strength, adaptability, and unwavering optimism.

Here's to your daily bravery, the healing power of food, and the bright life you live despite the hurdles. This book is for the genuine culinary fighters.

Table of Contents

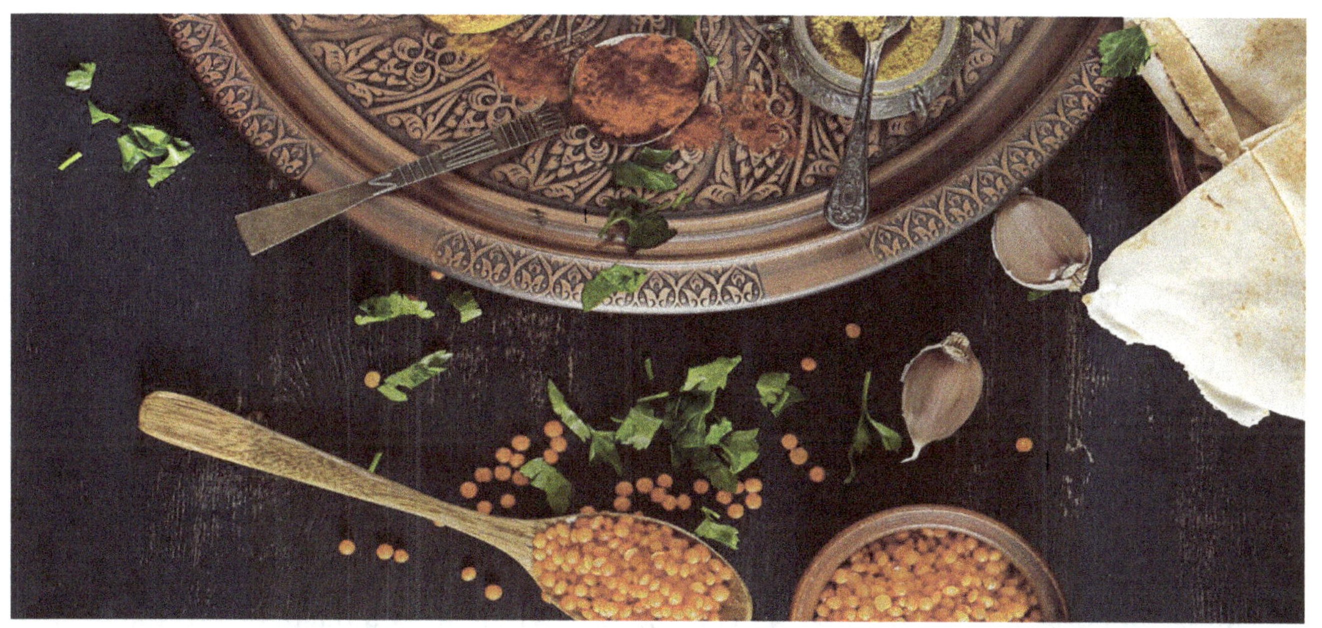

Introduction

Diverticulitis is not a sickness, but rather a condition in which small pouches called diverticula grow in the walls of the large intestine. These tiny pockets resemble hidden nooks where trouble could be lurking. When these pouches get inflamed, they cause diverticulitis, a dangerous ailment. Imagine your immune system as a watchful protector. When it detects trouble, it increases blood flow and dispatches disease-fighting cells to the area, resulting in inflammation. Suddenly, those harmless diverticula turn into a hub of activity.

Living with diverticulitis can be difficult, but your diet does not have to be monotonous or restricted. We think that eating should bring joy and sustenance, not worry. This cookbook is full of delectable, nutrient-dense meals that improve digestive health and reduce pain. We've done the research so you don't have to, developing meals that meet the dietary requirements of those with diverticulosis.

This cookbook is for anybody who has been diagnosed with diverticulosis and wishes to treat their symptoms via nutrition. It's also a great resource for family members, care-givers, and friends who are helping someone with diverticulosis.

Individuals diagnosed with diverticulosis: If you've been told to follow a certain diet to manage your disease, this book provides a treasure mine of recipes that adhere to medical restrictions while delighting your taste buds.

Family & Friends: Understanding someone's dietary preferences is essential while providing support for diverticulosis. This cookbook will help you make dishes that everyone will like, making sharing meals a pleasure rather than a chore.

Health enthusiasts: Even if you don't have diverticulosis, the concepts of a high-fiber, gut-friendly diet may help anybody who wants to enhance their digestion.

This cookbook will be a great choice as it includes the following:

- Bursting Flavors: Each recipe is designed to guarantee that you don't sacrifice flavor. Expect vivid, strong tastes that turn every meal into an experience.
- Nutritional Wisdom: Discover which foods are best for your condition, why they work, and how to integrate them into your diet with ease.
- Practical Tips: Learn how to plan meals, create shopping lists, and prepare using practices that will make your life easier and your digestive system happier.
- Diverse recipes: From substantial breakfasts and filling lunches to decadent evenings and tantalizing snacks, there's something for every taste and occasion.

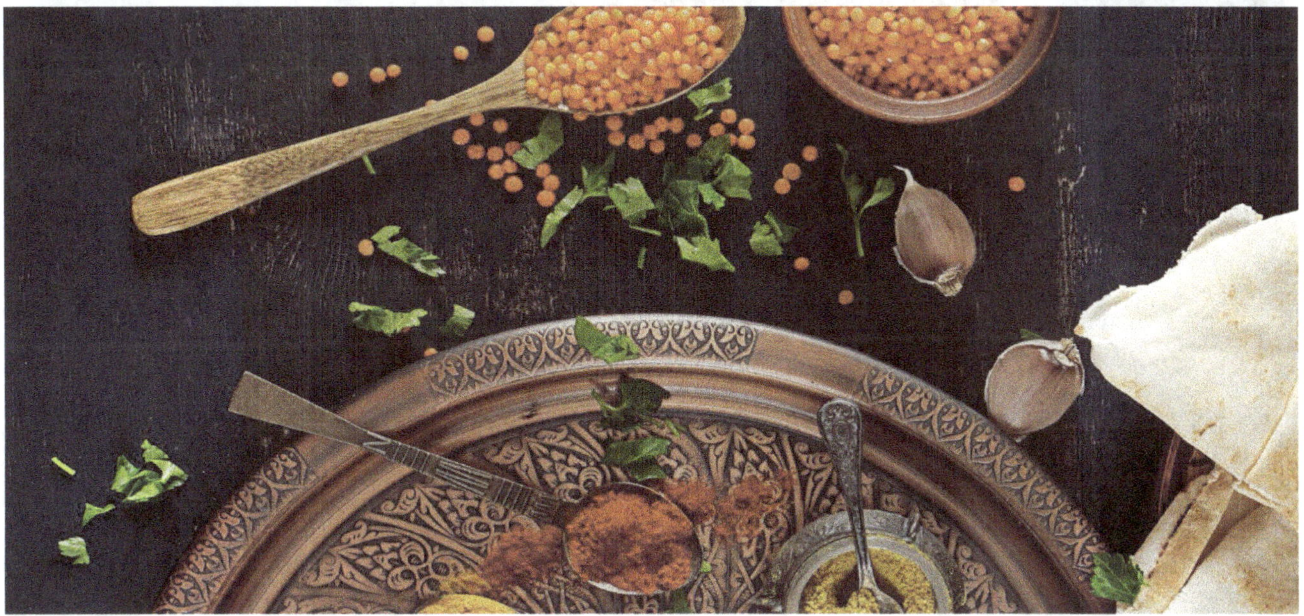

They can vary quite a little.

- Abdominal Pain: Typically felt on the lower left side, but can also occur on the right. The pain usually intensifies after eating and diminishes after having a bowel movement or passing gas.

- Digestive Changes: Your bowels may become constipated or diarrhoea as they play a guessing game. Blood in Stool: Occasionally, you may see blood in your stool, which is a clear indication that you should pay attention.

- Bloating: Your abdomen may feel bloated, like a balloon. If the inflammation becomes severe, you may experience:

- Persistent Abdominal discomfort: An ongoing, severe discomfort in your belly.

- Fever: Your body temperature may rise as your immune system fights back.

- Mucus in Stool: The presence of mucus in your stool can indicate severe irritation or inflammation.

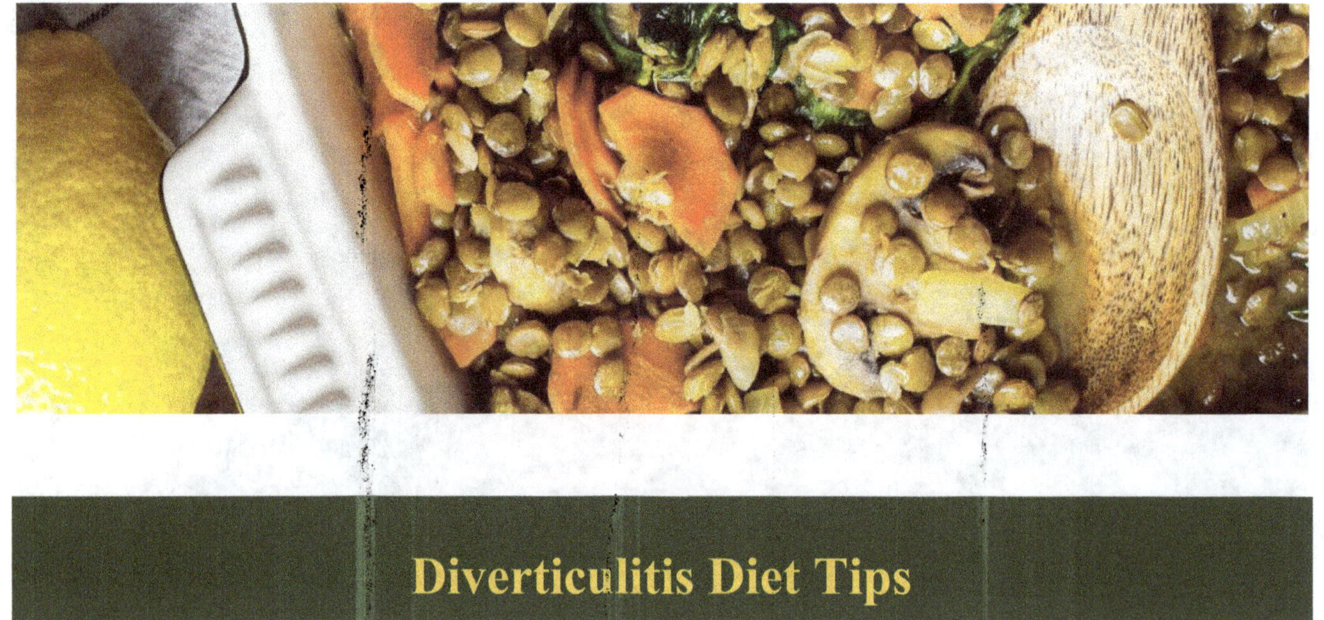

1) **Fibre Magic:** Dietary fibre, present in fruits, cereals, and vegetables, is critical. It bulks up stools, regulates bowel movements, and provides a smooth passage through the intestines. Without adequate fibre, faeces become hard and difficult to pass.

2) **Lifestyle changes:** Limit your use of alcohol, caffeine, aspirin, and non-steroidal anti-inflammatory medicines (such as ibuprofen). Exercise for 30 minutes, five days a week. Stop smoking to keep your intestines healthy. Maintain a healthy body-weight.

3) **Dietary delights:** Whole-Wheat Wonders: Eat whole-wheat bread, pasta, and cereal for a healthier colon.

4) **Bean Bonanza:** Eat kidney beans, black beans, and other legumes to improve intestinal health.

5) **Meat Moderation:** Limit red meat consumption (beef, hog, lamb) to 2-3 servings per week and have meat-free days twice a week.

6) **Fatty Foods:** Reduce your consumption of oily meals for a healthier colon.

BREAKFAST RECIPES

Oatmeal with Bananas

Ingredients:

- 1/2 cup old-fashioned oats (quick oats can also be used)
- 1 cup unsweetened almond milk (or any lactose-free milk)
- 1 ripe banana, sliced
- 1 tablespoon chopped walnuts (optional)
- Cinnamon (to taste)

Prep Time: 5 minutes

Instructions:

1. Cook the Muesli: In a saucepan, combine the oats and almond milk. Heat over medium-low heat, stirring occasionally, until the oats are completely cooked and the mixture thickens, which should take about 5 minutes.

2. Add the banana: Remove the pot from the heat and allow the muesli to cool slightly. Stir in the cut banana.

3. Optional toppings: If desired, add chopped walnuts for additional crunch and healthy fats. Add a dash of cinnamon for an added punch of flavour.

4. Serve warm. Divide the muesli into serving dishes and enjoy the cosy and nutritious muesli with bananas! Kilocalories Per

5. Serving: Approximately 250 calories (this can vary depending on the ingredients and portion size).

Spinach and Peeled Apple Smoothie

Ingredients:

- 1 cup fresh spinach leaves
- 1 peeled apple (cored and sliced)
- 1 cup water (or unsweetened almond milk)
- 1 teaspoon honey (optional, for sweetness)

Prep time	Kilocalories	Cooking	Total
5 minutes	80 kcal		

Instructions:

1. Rinse the spinach leaves thoroughly with cold water and pat dry.
2. Blend everything. In a blender, combine the spinach, diced peeled apple, water (or almond milk), and honey. Blend at high speeds until smooth and creamy.
3. To serve chilled, pour the spinach and peeled apple smoothie into a glass. Serve chilled and enjoy this delicious and gut-friendly beverage!

Egg Scramble with Sautéed Vegetables

Ingredients:

- 2 large eggs
- 1/2 cup chopped bell peppers (any color)
- 1/2 cup chopped spinach
- 1 teaspoon olive oil
- Salt and pepper to taste

Prep time	Kilo-calories per serving
10 Minutes	180

Instructions:

1. To sauté the veggies, heat olive oil in a nonstick skillet over medium heat. Sauté chopped bell peppers for 2-3 minutes, until slightly softened.
2. Add the chopped spinach and simmer for another 1-2 minutes, or until wilted. To scramble the eggs, crack them into a bowl and stir.
3. Pour the whisked eggs into the skillet among the sautéed veggies. Stir or scrape gently until the eggs are cooked and scrambled. Season with a pinch of salt and pepper.

4. Serve warm and enjoy your nutritious Egg Scramble with Sautéed Vegetables!

Whole Grain Cereal with Berries

<u>Ingredients:</u>

- 1/2 cup whole grain cereal (look for high-fiber options)
- 1/2 cup mixed berries (such as strawberries, blueberries, raspberries)
- 1 cup unsweetened almond milk (or any lactose-free milk)

Prep time	Kilocalories per ser
5 Minutes	200 kcal

<u>Instructions:</u>

1. Choose your cereal: Choose a whole grain cereal that has whole grains as the first ingredient (such as oats, bran, or quinoa). Check the label for fibre content.
2. Add berries: In a bowl, combine the cereal and mixed berries. You can use either fresh or frozen fruit.
3. Pour unsweetened almond milk (or lactose-free milk) over cereal and fruit.

4. Enjoy!: Mix everything together and enjoy your nutritious Whole Grain Cereal with Berries!

Whole Wheat Toast with Mashed Avocado

<u>Ingredients:</u>

- 1 slice whole wheat bread
- 1 ripe avocado
- Pinch of sea salt
- Optional: Black pepper or red pepper flakes

Prep time	Kilocalories per serving
5 minutes	200 kcal

<u>Instructions:</u>

1. Toast the whole wheat bread till crispy and golden. To mash the avocado, cut it in half, remove the seed, and scoop out the flesh in a dish.
2. Mash the avocado with a fork until it is creamy and smooth. To serve, generously spread mashed avocado on toasted bread.
3. Season and enjoy!: Sprinkle a pinch of sea salt on the avocado. If you want a

little kick, add some black pepper or red pepper flakes.

4. Serve your healthy whole wheat toast with mashed avocado while it's still warm.

Smoothie with Fruit, Leafy Greens and Flaxseed

Ingredients:

- 1 ripe banana
- 1 cup fresh spinach or kale (or a mix of both)
- 1 tablespoon ground flaxseed
- 1 cup water or unsweetened almond milk
- Ice cubes (optional, for extra chill)

Prep time	Kilocalories per serving
5 minutes	150 kcal

Instructions:

1. To make the smoothie, combine ripe banana, fresh spinach or kale, ground flaxseed, and water (or almond milk).

2. Blend until smooth. If you want your smoothie to be extremely cold, add a couple ice cubes. Blend until smooth.

Blend on high speed until thoroughly combined and smooth.

3. Serve and sip! Pour your smoothie with fruit, leafy greens, and flaxseed into a glass. Drink carefully and enjoy the goodness!

Greek Yogurt Parfait

Ingredients:

- 1 cup plain Greek yogurt
- 1/2 cup mixed berries (raspberries, blackberries, or blueberries)
- 1/4 cup granola (choose a low-sugar option)
- 1 tablespoon honey (optional, for sweetness)

Prep time	Kilocalories per serving
5 minutes	300 kcal

Instructions:

1. To layer Greek yoghurt, start by spooning it into the bottom of a glass or bowl.

2. Sprinkle oats on top of the Greek yoghurt. Layer fresh berries on top of

granola. Continue layering until the glass is full, then top with berries.

3. Drizzle with honey (optional). Drizzle a small quantity of honey over the parfait to give more sweetness.

4. Serve and enjoy!: Grab a spoon to enjoy the creamy yoghurt, crunchy granola, and juicy berries!

Chia Seed Pudding

Ingredients:

- 2 tablespoons chia seeds
- 1/2 cup almond milk (or any lactose-free milk)
- 1/2 teaspoon vanilla extract
- Optional: 1/2 cup diced mango or berries for topping

Prep time	Kilocalories per serving
5 minutes	150 kcal

Instructions:

1. Mix the ingredients. In a glass bowl or container, combine the chia seeds, almond milk, and vanilla essence. Stir thoroughly to mix.

2. Chill overnight. Cover the bowl or container and refrigerate. Allow it to gel overnight (or for at least four hours).

3. Check Consistency: Before serving, make sure the pudding is thickened and the chia seeds have gelled.

4. Top and enjoy!: Serve chia seed pudding with cream, coconut milk or fresh or frozen berries on top.

Buckwheat Pancakes

Ingredients:

- 1 cup buckwheat flour
- 1 teaspoon baking powder
- 1 tablespoon honey (optional, for sweetness)
- 1 cup almond milk (or any lactose-free milk)
- Cooking oil (for greasing the pan)

Prep time	Kilocalories per serving
10 minutes	200 kcl

1. To make the batter, combine buckwheat flour, baking powder, and almond milk. If you prefer your pancakes to be sweet, add honey.

2. Heat a nonstick frying pan on medium heat. Grease the pan with a bit of frying oil.

3. Cook the pancakes: Pour 2-3 teaspoons batter into the pan. Cook until bubbles appear on the surface (about 2-4 minutes). Flip and cook the other side until golden brown.

4. Serve warm. Stack your Buckwheat Pancakes and add your favourite toppings!

Quinoa Breakfast Bowl:

Ingredients:

- 1/2 cup cooked quinoa
- 1/2 cup mixed berries (such as strawberries, blueberries, raspberries)
- 1 tablespoon chopped nuts (such as

Prep time	Kilocalories per servings
10 minutes	250 kcl

almonds or walnuts)
- Optional: drizzle of honey for sweetness

Instructions:

1. Cook Quinoa: Prepare quinoa according to package directions (typically 1 part quinoa and 2 parts water).

2. Assemble the Bowl. In a bowl, arrange the cooked quinoa. Garnish with mixed berries and chopped nuts.

3. Sweeten (optional): If you want to add some sweetness, drizzle with honey.

4. Enjoy!: Mix everything together and enjoy your nutritious Quinoa Breakfast Bowl!

02

Turkey and Quinoa Stuffed Peppers

Ingredients:

- 1 cup cooked quinoa
- 4 oz ground turkey
- Bell peppers (red, yellow, or green), halved
- Tomato sauce (low sodium)
- Italian herbs for seasoning

Prep time	Kiloalories per servings
15 minutes	350 kcl

Instructions:

1. Cook the quinoa: Prepare quinoa according to package directions (typically 1 part quinoa and 2 parts water). Cook the ground turkey in a pan until browned.
2. Combine Quinoa and Turkey: In a bowl, combine the cooked quinoa and the browned turkey. Season with Italian herbs.
3. Stuff the peppers: Fill the bell pepper halves with the turkey-quinoa mixture. To bake, place the filled peppers in a baking dish. Pour the tomato sauce over the top.
4. Bake at 375°F (190°C) for about 20 minutes, or until the peppers are soft. Serve warm.
5. Enjoy the soothing Turkey and Quinoa Stuffed Peppers!

Lentil and Vegetable Soup

Ingredients:

- 1 cup dried green or brown lentils
- 2 carrots, diced
- 2 celery stalks, chopped
- 1 onion, diced
- 4 cups low-sodium vegetable broth
- 1 teaspoon dried thyme
- Salt and pepper to taste

Prep time	Kilocalories per servings
15 minutes	50 kcl

Instructions:

1. Rinse lentils with cool water. To sauté vegetables, cook diced carrots, celery, and onion until softened.

2. Add washed lentils and veggie broth to the pot. Season with dried thyme, salt, and pepper.

3. Simmer: Bring soup to a boil, then reduce heat and simmer for 30 minutes or until lentils are cooked.

4. To serve warm, ladle the lentil and vegetable soup into bowls. Enjoy your hearty, gut-friendly soup!

Salmon Salad Wraps

Ingredients:

- 1 can of salmon (drained and skin removed)
- 1/2 cucumber (diced)
- 1 celery stalk (chopped)
- 1/4 red onion (finely chopped)
- 2 tablespoons plain Greek yogurt
- Salt and pepper to taste
- Collard green leaves (for wrapping)

Prep time	Kilocalories per servings
10 minutes	200 kcal

Instructions:

1. Mix the salad: In a bowl, combine the drained salmon, diced cucumber, celery, and finely chopped red onion.

2. Season with salt and pepper after adding the plain Greek yoghurt.

3. Assemble the Wraps Lay out the collard green leaves. Spoon some salmon salad onto each leaf.

4. Roll and enjoy! Roll the collard green leaves into a wrap. Secure with toothpicks if necessary.

5. Enjoy your delicious and nutritious Salmon Salad Wraps!

Chickpea and Spinach Curry

Ingredients:

- 1 can of chickpeas (drained and rinsed)
- 2 cups fresh baby spinach
- 1 onion (chopped)
- 2 garlic cloves (minced)
- 1 teaspoon ground cumin
- 1 teaspoon ground coriander
- 1/2 teaspoon turmeric
- 1/4 teaspoon cayenne pepper (adjust to taste)
- 1 can of chopped tomatoes

- Salt and pepper to taste
- Optional: Fresh cilantro for garnish

Prep time	Kilocalories per servings
15 minutes	250 kcal

Instructions:

1. To sauté onion and garlic, heat some oil in a pan. Combine the chopped onion and minced garlic. Sauté until soft. Stir in ground cumin, coriander, turmeric, and cayenne pepper.
2. Add drained chickpeas and canned chopped tomatoes.
3. Season with salt and pepper. Simmer curry for 10 minutes, stirring occasionally. Add fresh baby spinach to the curry.
4. Cook until wilted. Serve warm and garnish with fresh cilantro if preferred.
5. Enjoy your comforting Chickpea and Spinach Curry!

Quinoa and Black Bean Salad

Ingredients:

- 1 cup cooked quinoa
- 1 can of black beans (drained and rinsed)
- 1 red bell pepper (diced)
- 1/2 red onion (finely chopped)
- Fresh cilantro (chopped, to taste)
- Juice of 1 lime
- Salt and pepper to taste

Prep time	Kilocalories per servings
15 minutes	300 kcal

Instructions:

1. In a large mixing bowl, combine cooked quinoa, black beans, diced red bell pepper, finely chopped red onion, and fresh cilantro.
2. To add lime juice, squeeze one lime over the salad. Season with salt and pepper to taste.
3. To serve chilled, toss all ingredients thoroughly.
4. Serve your Quinoa and Black Bean Salad cold!

Chicken and Vegetable Stir-Fry

Ingredients:

- 1 boneless, skinless chicken breast (sliced)
- 1 red bell pepper (sliced)
- 1 zucchini (sliced)
- 1 carrot (julienned)
- 2 cloves of garlic (minced)
- 1 tablespoon olive oil
- Low-sodium soy sauce (to taste)

Prep time	Kilocalories per sevings
15 minutes	300 kcal

Instructions:

1. To sauté chicken, heat olive oil in a pan over medium high heat. Combine the sliced chicken and minced garlic.
2. Cook the chicken until it is no longer pink. To add veggies, add sliced red pepper, zucchini and julienned carrot to the pan.
3. Stir-fry for about 5-7 minutes, until the vegetables are soft and crisp. Season chicken and vegetables with low-sodium soy sauce. Season with salt and pepper to taste.
4. Serve warm. Enjoy your colourful and gut-friendly chicken and vegetables. Stir-Fry!

Greek Yogurt Tuna Salad

Ingredients:

- 1 can of tuna (drained)
- 1/2 cup plain Greek yogurt
- 1 celery stalk (diced)
- 1/4 red onion (finely chopped)
- 1 teaspoon Dijon mustard
- Salt and pepper to taste

Prep time	Kilocalories per servings
5 minutes	200 kcal

Instructions

1. To make the salad, combine drained tuna, plain Greek yoghurt, diced celery, finely chopped red onion, and Dijon mustard.
2. Mix everything thoroughly until fully blended. Season with salt and pepper to taste.

3. Serve and enjoy!: Serve creamy Greek Yoghurt Tuna Salad with whole-grain crackers, toast, salad leaves, or tortillas.

Sweet Potato and Lentil Bowl

Ingredients:

- 1 cup cooked green or brown lentils
- 1 medium sweet potato (peeled and cubed)
- 1 cup baby spinach
- 1/4 red onion (finely chopped)
- Olive oil (for roasting sweet potatoes)
- Salt and pepper to taste

Prep time	Kilocalories per servings
20 minute	300 kcal

Instructions:

1. Roast sweet potatoes: Preheat the oven to 400 °F (200 °C). Toss the diced sweet potatoes with olive oil, salt, and pepper. Roast in the oven for about 15-20 minutes, until tender.

2. Assemble the Bowl In a bowl, combine cooked lentils, roasted sweet potatoes, baby spinach, and finely sliced red onion. To season, drizzle with extra olive oil as required.

3. Season with salt and pepper to taste. S

4. erve warm. Enjoy this nutritious Sweet Potato and Lentil Bowl!

Zucchini Noodles with Pesto

Ingredients:

- 2 medium zucchinis (about 500g), spiralized into noodles
- 2 tablespoons olive oil
- 1/4 cup sunflower seeds or pine nuts (for the pesto)
- 1/2 cup grated Parmesan cheese (or vegan Parmesan)
- 2 cloves of garlic, minced
- Salt, to taste
- Splash of unsweetened almond milk (about 2 tablespoons)

Nutritional Information (per serving):
Calories: Approximately 226 kcal
Net Carbs: Less than 2 grams

Instructions:

1. Prepare the zucchini noodles: Wash the zucchinis and remove the skin with a vegetable peeler.

2. Use a spiralizer or mandolin to make spaghetti-like strands. The spiralizer is great for creating consistent noodles.

3. To eliminate any extra moisture, pat dry the zucchini noodles with a paper towel.

4. Cook the zucchini noodles: Preheat a lightly greased frying pan over medium heat. Stir-fry the zucchini noodles for about 5 minutes, until they soften and become slightly crunchy. Remove from the pan and set aside.

5. Make the pesto: In a food processor or blender, add sunflower seeds (or pine nuts), minced garlic, grated Parmesan cheese, and a touch of salt. Blend until your pesto sauce is smooth. If necessary, add a splash of unsweetened almond milk to achieve the desired consistency.

6. Combine and serve. Return the cooked zucchini noodles to the pan. Toss in the pesto sauce, making sure the noodles are completely coated.

7. Serve warm, with more Parmesan cheese if desired.

Eggplant and Quinoa Bake

Ingredients:

- 1 leek (about 1 cup), sliced and cleaned
- 1 small head of cauliflower (about 4 cups), chopped into bite-sized pieces
- 4 small eggplants (about 4 cups), medium diced, sprinkled with salt and drained on a paper towel
- 1 can (15 oz) artichoke hearts, drained and halved
- 1 cup almond milk
- 2 cups plain yogurt
- 1 tablespoon dried oregano
- 1 teaspoon nutmeg
- 4 cups spinach
- 4 cups quinoa, cooked
- Salt and pepper, to taste
- 1 cup low-fat mozzarella cheese, shredded

<u>**Instructions:**</u>

1. Prepare the vegetables. In a sauté pan, heat the olive oil over medium-high heat. Add the leeks and sweat for about 2 minutes, or until they become translucent. Combine the cauliflower, eggplant, and artichokes.

2. Stir to mix. Season to taste with salt and pepper, cover, and simmer for approximately 20 minutes, or until the veggies are tender. If the pan appears to be too dry, add approximately 1/4 cup of water.

3. Make the yoghurt mixture: In a medium-sized bowl, combine almond milk and yoghurt. Combine the dried oregano and nutmeg. Combine the spinach and cooked quinoa in the yoghurt mixture.

4. Mix well. Taste for salt and pepper. Assembly and Baking: Preheat your oven to 350°F (180°C). Pour the vegetable and quinoa mixture into a baking dish.

5. Top with shredded mozzarella cheese. Bake in the preheated oven for 15 minutes, or until the cheese on top has lightly browned. Serve warm and allow to cool slightly before serving. Enjoy this warm and nutritious Eggplant and Quinoa Bake!

Nutritional Information (per serving):
Calories: Approximately 298 kcal
Fat: 16 g
Saturated Fat: 6 g
Carbohydrates: 29 g
Sugar: 5 g
Fiber: 7 g
Protein: 14 g
Sodium: 722 mg

03

STEW RECIPES

French Oven Beef Stew

Ingredients:

- 1 kg (2.2 lbs) onions, sliced
- 2 kg (4.4 lbs) chuck steak, cut into 6–7 cm (2.4–2.8 inches) chunks
- 4–5 fresh thyme or oregano sprigs
- 2 bay leaves
- 5 cloves of garlic, chopped or sliced (about 25g)
- 100 ml (3.4 fl oz) olive oil
- Zest of 1 orange
- 750 ml (25.4 fl oz) Côtes du Rhône red wine
- 750 ml (25.4 fl oz) beef stock
- 200 g (7 oz) bacon lardons
- Salt and white pepper

Instructions:

1. Marinate the stew. Mix the onions, chuck steak, thyme or oregano sprigs, bay leaves, garlic, olive oil, orange zest, and Côtes du Rhône red wine in a bowl. Season with white pepper.

2. Allow to marinate for 24 hours. Slowly Cook the Stew: Preheat the oven to 150°C (300°F), or Fan 130°C (266°F). Pour all of the marinade into a flameproof casserole dish. Bring to a simmer on the stove, then transfer the dish to the oven.

3. Cook for 4 hours, or until the beef is meltingly soft. Add beef stock and lardons. Remove from the oven and allow to cool.

4. Refrigerate overnight. The following day, preheat the oven to 150°C (300°F) or Fan 130°C (266°F). Add the beef stock and bacon lardons to the stew.

5. Bring to a simmer on the hob, as before. Place the casserole back in the oven and cook for another two hours.

6. Serve warm. Discard the bay leaves. Enjoy your thick, delicious French Oven Beef Stew!

Nutritional Information (per serving):
Calories: Approximately 248 kcal
Fat: 37 g

Chicken and Vegetable Stew

Ingredients:

- 1 lb boneless, skinless chicken breasts (or boneless, skinless chicken thighs)
- 4 medium russet potatoes, peeled and diced
- 1 bag (about 16 oz) frozen mixed vegetables (peas, carrots, corn, and green beans)
- 1 large onion, chopped
- 3 cloves of garlic, minced
- 2 sprigs of fresh thyme
- 1 sprig of fresh rosemary
- 4 cups chicken stock (use stock for richer flavor)
- 1/2 cup heavy cream
- 2 tablespoons vegetable oil
- 2 tablespoons butter
- 2 tablespoons all-purpose flour
- Salt and pepper, to taste

Instructions:

1. To brown the chicken, heat vegetable oil and butter in a large soup pot on medium heat. Add the chicken and cook on both sides.

2. Remove the chicken from the pot and set it aside. Sauté the aromatics in the same saucepan with chopped onions and minced garlic. Sauté the onions until they're tender and aromatic.

3. Add the fresh thyme and rosemary sprigs. To deglaze the pot, add chicken stock and cook over high heat. Use a whisk to scrape off any browned bits from the pot's bottom. Add diced potatoes and frozen mixed vegetables to the saucepan.

4. Simmer for approximately 15 minutes, or until the potatoes are soft and the mixture thickens. To finish the dish, cut the browned chicken into bite-sized pieces and return to the pot.

5. To achieve a silky texture, stir in the heavy cream. Season with salt and pepper to taste.

6. To serve warm, remove the thyme and rosemary sprigs. Enjoy this nourishing Chicken and Vegetable Stew!

Nutritional Information (per serving):

Calories: Approximately 415 kcal

Protein: 48 g

Carbohydrates: 26.5 g

Sugars: 7.5 g

Fat: 11 g

Saturated Fat: 2 g

Fiber: 8 g

Sodium: 0.5 g

Lentil and Spinach Stew

Ingredients:

- 2 tablespoons olive oil
- 1 large onion, finely chopped
- 3 cloves of garlic, minced
- 2 teaspoons ground cumin
- 1 teaspoon crushed red pepper (adjust to taste)
- 1 cup small brown lentils, rinsed and prepared
- 4 cups vegetable broth
- 10 oz (300g) fresh spinach, loosely packed
- Salt and pepper, to taste

Instructions:

1. To sauté aromatics, heat olive oil in a medium saucepan over medium heat. Cook until the onion is transparent, about 3-5 minutes.

2. Combine minced garlic, ground cumin, and crushed red pepper. Cook until aromatic, about 1 minute.

3. To prepare the lentils and broth, rinse them and add them to a saucepan. Add the vegetable broth and bring to a boil.

4. Cook the lentils until they are soft (approximately 20 minutes). Stir in fresh spinach leaves. Allow them to wilt into the stew.

5. Season and serve with salt and pepper to taste. Serve warm with good bread.

Nutritional Information (per serving):

Calories: Approximately 248 kcal

Protein: 14 g

Carbohydrates: 38 g

Fiber: 12 g

Fat: 6 g

Iron: 4 mg

Ingredients:

- 4 tablespoons extra virgin olive oil
- 1 large onion, thinly sliced
- 1 green bell pepper, thinly sliced
- 1 yellow bell pepper, thinly sliced
- 2 garlic cloves, minced
- 1 stalk celery, diced
- 2 carrots, peeled and thinly sliced
- 1 sweet potato, peeled and cut into 1-inch cubes
- 2 lbs (about 900 g) skinless, boneless turkey thighs or breasts, cut into 1-inch pieces
- 1 (28 oz) can Red Gold® Whole Peeled Tomatoes (or 2 cans of 14.5 oz each)
- 1 tablespoon Hungarian sweet paprika
- Salt and black pepper, to taste
- 1/4 teaspoon cayenne pepper
- 1 tablespoon Worcestershire sauce
- 1 tablespoon lemon juice
- 1 teaspoon chopped fresh rosemary
- 2 teaspoons cornstarch
- 3/4 cup plain yogurt

Instructions:

1. In a large Dutch oven or pot, heat the olive oil. Sauté the onion, bell peppers, garlic, celery, and carrots until tender. Combine sweet potatoes, turkey, Red Gold Whole Peeled Tomatoes, paprika, salt, pepper, cayenne, Worcestershire sauce, lemon juice, and rosemary.

2. Cover and heat until the turkey is done and the sweet potatoes are soft (approximately 30-40 minutes).

3. To thicken the stew, mix cornflour with a little water and toss it in. Serve with a spoonful of plain yoghurt. Enjoy!

White Bean and Kale Stew

Ingredients:

- 3 tablespoons olive oil
- 1 medium onion, diced
- 3 cloves fresh garlic, minced
- 1/4 cup dry white wine
- 14.5 oz. canned Italian tomatoes, diced
- 3 cups cannellini beans (canned is fine)
- 2 cups vegetable broth
- 1/2 medium lemon
- 1-2 cups fresh kale, chopped
- 2 tablespoons fresh parsley
- 1 teaspoon salt
- 1/2 teaspoon pepper
- 1 loaf fresh bread (optional, for making bruschetta)

Instructions:

1. Heat the olive oil in a big, deep skillet or saucepan over medium heat. Add the diced onion and sauté for 5 minutes. Cook for a further 1 minute after adding the garlic.
2. Add the white wine, scraping off any onion and garlic crumbs. Add the tinned tomatoes and cannellini beans, and cook for 3 minutes. Add the veggie broth, lemon juice, and kale. Cook for another 5 minutes.
3. Mash part of the beans using a potato masher or a sturdy spoon. Season with parsley, salt, and pepper, to taste. Save some parsley for garnish.
4. Serve heated as a stew or with fresh bread for bruschetta.

Salmon Chowder

Ingredients:

- 2-3 tablespoons olive oil or butter
- 1 onion, diced
- 1 small fennel bulb, diced
- 1 cup celery, diced
- 2-4 garlic cloves, minced
- 1 teaspoon fennel seeds
- ½ teaspoon thyme
- ½ teaspoon smoked paprika
- ⅓ cup white wine
- 3 cups chicken broth
- ¾ lb baby red potatoes, sliced thin
- Salt and pepper, to taste
- 1 bay leaf
- 1 lb salmon, cooked and flaked (no skin/bones)
- 1 cup heavy cream

1. To sauté aromatics, cook onion, fennel bulb, and celery in olive oil or butter on medium heat.

2. Add the minced garlic, thyme, fennel seeds, and smoked paprika.

3. Mix in white wine and chicken broth. Add the bay leaf and bring to a simmer over high heat. Add the cut potatoes.

4. Cook until tender. Reduce the heat to medium-low and cook the potatoes until they are soft.

5. Finish the chowder: Stir in the heavy cream, followed by the cooked and flaked salmon.

6. Remove from heat. To season and garnish, add salt and pepper to taste. Garnish with lemon slices and fennel fronds.

7. Serve and Enjoy! Ladle into bowls and enjoy this delectable Salmon Chowder!

Mushroom and Barley Stew

Ingredients:

- 2 onions
- 1 leek
- 2 carrots
- 400g chestnut mushrooms
- 3 garlic cloves
- A handful of thyme leaves (leaves only)
- 1 glass of white wine
- 1 liter hot chicken or vegetable stock
- 150g pearl barley
- 150ml double cream

Instructions:

1. Prepare the vegetables. Peel and thinly slice the carrots and onions. Trim, clean, and slice the leek thinly. Tear the mushrooms into small pieces. Peel and slice the garlic.

2. Pick and coarsely cut the thyme leaves. Sauté the vegetables. In a large pan, heat 1 tablespoon oil over medium heat. Combine the onions, leeks, carrots, mushrooms, garlic, and thyme. Season with salt and pepper.

3. Cook for 12-15 minutes, stirring periodically, until the veggies have

softened. Add wine and stock. Turn up the heat to high and pour in a glass of white wine.

4. Bring to a boil, then decrease the wine by half. Combine 1 litre of chicken or vegetable stock with 150g of pearl barley.

5. Bring to a boil again, then lower to a simmer. Cover and cook for 35-40 minutes, until the barley is cooked.

6. Finish and serve. Stir in 150ml of double cream and heat thoroughly. Ladle into bowls and enjoy your delicious Mushroom and Barley Stew!

Nutritional Information (per serving):

Calories: Approximately 248 kcal

Total Fat: 16 g

Saturated Fat: 10 g

Cholesterol: 48 mg

Sodium: 28 mg

Carbohydrates: 24 g

Fiber: 4 g

Protein: 4 g

Tomato and Quinoa Stew

Ingredients:

- 1 cup quinoa
- 2 cups water
- 1 tablespoon olive oil
- 1 onion, chopped
- 2 cloves of garlic, minced
- 1 teaspoon dried basil
- 1 teaspoon dried oregano
- 1 can (28 oz) fire-roasted tomatoes
- 2 cups vegetable broth
- Salt and pepper, to taste
- Fresh basil leaves (for garnish)

Instructions:

1. Cook the Quinoa

2. Rinse the quinoa under cold water. In a saucepan, combine quinoa and water. Bring to a boil, then reduce heat and simmer for 15 minutes or until quinoa is cooked and water is absorbed.

3. Sauté Aromatics: Heat olive oil in a large pot over medium heat. Add chopped onion and minced garlic. Sauté until softened.

4. Add Tomatoes and Spices: Stir in dried basil and oregano. Add fire-

roasted tomatoes (with their juices) and vegetable broth. Season with salt and pepper.

5. Simmer and Combine: Simmer for 10-15 minutes to allow flavors to meld. Add cooked quinoa to the pot and stir to combine.

6. Serve & Enjoy!

7. Ladle into bowls, garnish with fresh basil leaves, and savor this wholesome Tomato and Quinoa Stew!

Nutritional Information (per serving):

Calories: Approximately 220 kcal

Protein: 7 g

Carbohydrates: 38 g

Fiber: 6 g

Fat: 5 g

Vegetable and Chickpea Stew

Ingredients:

- 1 red onion, chopped
- 3 cloves of garlic, minced
- 1 teaspoon ground cumin
- 1 teaspoon smoked paprika
- 2 medium carrots, peeled and diced
- 2 medium sweet potatoes, peeled and diced
- 1 can (14 oz) diced tomatoes
- 1 can (14 oz) chickpeas (garbanzo beans), drained and rinsed
- 4 cups vegetable broth
- Salt and pepper, to taste
- Fresh parsley or cilantro (for garnish)

Instructions:

1. Sauté Aromatics: Heat olive oil in a big pot on medium heat. Combine the chopped red onion and minced garlic. Sauté until soft. Add spices and vegetables. Stir in the ground cumin and smoked paprika.

2. Combine the diced carrots and sweet potatoes. Pour in the canned diced tomatoes (with the liquids). Simmer and combine. Combine the drained chickpeas and vegetable broth. Season with salt and pepper.

3. Bring to a simmer and cook until the vegetables are soft, about 20-25 minutes. Serve and Enjoy! Ladle into bowls, top with fresh parsley or

cilantro, and enjoy this nutritious Vegetable and Chickpea Stew!

Nutritional Information (per serving):

Calories: Approximately 220 kcal

Protein: 8 g

Carbohydrates: 45 g

Fiber: 10 g

Fat: 2 g

Sweet Corn and Potato Stew

Ingredients:

- 2 medium sweet potatoes, peeled and diced
- 1 medium red onion, chopped
- 2 cloves of garlic, minced
- 2 cups fresh or frozen sweet corn kernels
- 4 cups vegetable broth
- 1 teaspoon ground cumin
- Salt and pepper, to taste
- Fresh parsley or cilantro (for garnish)

Instructions:

1. Sauté Aromatics: Heat olive oil in a big pot on medium heat. Combine the chopped red onion and minced garlic. Sauté until soft.
2. Add Sweet Potatoes and Corn: Combine the diced sweet potatoes and sweet corn kernels. Pour in the veggie broth. Season with ground cumin, salt, and pepper.
3. Simmer and combine. Bring the stew to a simmer and cook until the sweet potatoes are cooked, about 20 minutes.
4. Serve and Enjoy! Ladle into bowls, sprinkle with fresh parsley or cilantro, and enjoy this nutritious Sweet Corn and Potato Stew!

Nutritional Information (per serving):

Calories: Approximately 220 kcal

Protein: 4 g

Carbohydrates: 50 g

Fiber: 6 g

Fat: 1 g

04

Grilled Chicken with White Rice and Steamed Carrots

Ingredients:

- 2 boneless, skinless chicken breasts
- 1 cup white rice
- 2 cups water
- 2 large carrots, peeled and sliced
- Olive oil
- Salt and pepper, to taste
- Fresh parsley (for garnish)

Instructions:

1. To prepare the grill, preheat it to medium-high heat. You can use an outdoor grill or a stove-top grill pan.

2. Marinate chicken (optional): Marinate the chicken breasts in your favourite herbs and spices for added flavour. Lemon juice, garlic, rosemary, and thyme all work well. Grill the chicken breasts for 3-4 minutes per side, according on thickness. Flip the chicken 2-3 times while cooking to promote equal browning.

3. Cook the white rice: Rinse the white rice with cool water. In a saucepan, mix the rinsed rice with 2 cups of water. Bring to a boil, then reduce the heat and simmer for 15 minutes, or until the rice is cooked and the water has been absorbed. Steam sliced carrots in a separate saucepan until soft (5-7 minutes).

4. Serve and Enjoy! Plate the grilled chicken with white rice and steamed vegetables. Drizzle with olive oil, season with salt and pepper, and finish with fresh parsley.

Nutritional Information (per serving):

Calories: Approximately 350 kcal

Protein: 30 g

Carbohydrates: 40 g

Fiber: 4 g

Fat: 8 g

Baked Cod with Mashed Potatoes and Green Beans

Ingredients:

- 2 large russet potatoes, scrubbed, sliced thin or cubed (about 2 lbs.)
- 4 tablespoons extra-virgin olive oil, divided
- Kosher salt
- Freshly ground black pepper
- 4 (6-ounce) cod or other meaty white fish fillets
- 1 pound fresh or frozen green beans
- ½ cup caramelized onions (about 2 onions)

Instructions:

1. Preheating the oven: Set the oven temperature to 220°C (200°C fan/gas mark 7).
2. To prepare the potatoes and green beans: In a roasting pan, combine the lemon wedges, chorizo, and tomatoes. Bake for 10 minutes. Pour the wine over the fish fillets in the container.
3. Season generously, then wrap the tray tightly with kitchen foil. Steam bake the salmon for 10 minutes, or until fully cooked.
4. Serve and relish: Place the baked cod next to the mashed potatoes and green beans. Drizzle with olive oil, sprinkle with salt and pepper, then top with caramelised onions.

Nutritional Information (per serving):
Calories: Approximately 400 kcal
Protein: 30 g
Carbohydrates: 40 g
Fiber: 8 g
Fat: 15 g

Scrambled Eggs with Toast and Fruit Juice

Ingredients:

- 2 large eggs
- 1 tablespoon butter
- Salt and pepper, to taste
- 2 slices whole-grain bread (toasted)
- 1 cup fruit juice (such as orange or apple)

Instructions:

1. To prepare the eggs, crack them into a basin and whisk until thoroughly blended. Season with a pinch of salt and pepper.

2. Cook the eggs: Melt the butter in a nonstick skillet over medium-low heat. Pour in the whisked eggs and allow it settle for a few seconds.

3. Gently whisk the eggs with a spatula, pushing them from the sides to the centre. Continue to mix until the eggs are soft and creamy (approximately 1-2 minutes). Toast whole grain bread while eggs boil.

4. Serve and Enjoy: Place the scrambled eggs on the toasted bread. Pour a glass of fruit juice to the side.

Nutritional Information (per serving):

Calories: Approximately 275 kcal

Protein: 17 g

Carbohydrates: 20 g

Fat: 14 g

Salmon Salad with Avocado and Quinoa

Ingredients:

- 2 salmon fillets
- 1 cup quinoa
- 2 cups chicken stock
- 1 ripe avocado, peeled, seeded, and coarsely chopped
- 1 cup halved cherry tomatoes
- 1/2 cucumber, diced
- 1/4 red onion, finely chopped
- Fresh basil leaves (for garnish)
- Olive oil
- Salt and pepper, to taste

Instructions:

1. To cook the salmon: Sprinkle the salmon fillets with salt and pepper. Grill or pan-sear the salmon until it reaches your desired level of doneness. Slice the salmon into bite-sized chunks.

2. Cooking the Quinoa: Rinse the quinoa under cool water. In a saucepan, combine the rinsed quinoa with 2 cups of chicken broth. Bring to a boil, then reduce to a simmer for 15 minutes, or

until the quinoa is cooked and the liquid has been absorbed.

3. To assemble the salad: In a large mixing bowl, add the cooked quinoa, avocado, cherry tomatoes, cucumber, and red onion. Drizzle olive oil and season with salt and pepper.

4. Toss gently until combined. Serve & enjoy! Plate the quinoa salad and garnish with the grilled salmon pieces. Garnish with basil leaves.

Nutritional Information (per serving):

Calories: Approximately 400 kcal

Protein: 30 g

Carbohydrates: 40 g

Fiber: 8 g

Fat: 15 g

Turkey Meatballs with Zucchini Noodles

Ingredients:

- 1 pound ground turkey
- 1/2 cup Panko breadcrumbs
- 1/4 cup freshly grated Parmesan cheese
- 2 large egg yolks
- 1 teaspoon dried oregano
- 1 teaspoon dried basil
- 1/2 teaspoon dried parsley
- 1/4 teaspoon garlic powder
- 1/4 teaspoon crushed red pepper flakes
- Salt and freshly ground black pepper, to taste
- 3 medium-sized zucchinis, spiralized
- 2 teaspoons salt
- 2 cups marinara sauce (homemade or store-bought)
- 1/4 cup freshly grated Parmesan cheese

Instructions:

1. Preheat the Oven: Set your oven to 400°F (200°C). Lightly oil or spray a 9×13 baking dish.

2. Make the Turkey Meatballs: In a large bowl, mix together ground turkey, Panko breadcrumbs, grated Parmesan, egg yolks, oregano, basil, parsley, garlic powder, crushed red pepper, salt, and pepper. Roll into 1 1/2- to 2-inch meatballs (about 24) and place them in the baking dish.

3. Bake the Meatballs: Bake for 18-20 minutes, until browned and cooked through. Set aside.

4. Prepare the Zucchini Noodles: Spiralize the zucchini and place it in a strainer over the sink. Sprinkle with salt and mix gently. Let sit for 10 minutes. Sauté the zucchini in boiling water for 30 seconds to 1 minute. Drain well.

5. Assemble the Dish: Divide the zucchini noodles into meal prep containers. Top with turkey meatballs, marinara sauce, and grated Parmesan.

6. Serve and Enjoy: Enjoy this light, healthy, and low-carb meal!

Nutritional Information (per serving):

Calories: Approximately 400 kcal

Protein: 30 g

Carbohydrates: 40 g

Fiber: 8 g

Fat: 15 g

Vegetable Stir-Fry with Tofu

Ingredients:

- 1 block of extra-firm tofu, pressed and cubed
- 2 tablespoons vegetable oil
- 1 red bell pepper, sliced
- 1 yellow bell pepper, sliced
- 1 medium zucchini, sliced
- 1 cup broccoli florets
- 1 cup snap peas
- 2 cloves garlic, minced
- 1 tablespoon fresh ginger, grated
- 3 tablespoons low-sodium soy sauce
- 1 tablespoon cornstarch
- 1 tablespoon water
- 1 teaspoon sesame oil
- 1 teaspoon rice vinegar

- 1 teaspoon honey (optional)
- Sesame seeds (for garnish)
- Green onions (for garnish)

Instructions:

1. Prepare the tofu: Press the tofu to remove any excess water. Cut into bite-size bits.

2. Stir fry the tofu: Heat 1 tablespoon vegetable oil in a large wok or skillet over medium-high heat. Cook until the tofu is golden brown on all sides. Remove and set aside.

3. Stir fry the vegetables: In the same pan, heat an additional tablespoon of vegetable oil. Include sliced bell peppers, zucchini, broccoli, and snap peas. Stir-fry for 3-4 minutes, until the vegetables are soft and crisp. Cook for another 30 seconds, then add the minced garlic and grated ginger.

4. Make the sauce: In a small bowl, combine the soy sauce, cornflour, water, sesame oil, rice vinegar, and honey (if using). Combine everything. Return the tofu to the pan alongside the vegetables. Pour the sauce over the tofu and vegetables. Toss until everything is equally covered and heated through.

5. Serve and enjoy. Serve the stir-fry hot, topped with sesame seeds and green onions.

Nutritional Information (per serving):

Calories: Approximately 250 kcal

Protein: 15 g

Carbohydrates: 20 g

Fiber: 5 g

Fat: 12 g

Baked Sweet Potato with Cottage Cheese and Chives

Ingredients:

- 1 medium sweet potato (about 350g/12oz), washed and dried
- 2 tbsp olive oil
- 1/2 cup low-fat cottage cheese
- Fresh chives, chopped
- Salt and pepper, to taste

Instructions:

1. Preheat the oven. Preheat the oven to 400 °F (200 °C). Prepare the sweet potato: Cut the raw sweet potato in half lengthwise.
2. Drizzle the halves with olive oil, then rub it into the skins and flesh. Place the halves, cut sides facing down, on a baking sheet.
3. Bake the sweet potatoes: Bake until the sweet potatoes are fork-tender (approximately 25 to 30 minutes). Let the pan cool for a few minutes.
4. Assemble the dish Flip the halves over and season with salt and pepper. Top each sweet potato half with a big scoop of low-fat cottage cheese. Garnish with freshly chopped chives.
5. Serve and Enjoy! Enjoy this balanced and healthful baked sweet potato with cottage cheese and chives!

Nutritional Information (per serving):

Calories: Approximately 250 kcal

Protein: 10 g

Carbohydrates: 40 g

Fiber: 6 g

Fat: 6 g

Quinoa-Stuffed Bell Peppers

Ingredients:

- 4 large bell peppers (any color)
- 1 cup quinoa, rinsed
- 2 cups vegetable broth
- 1 can (15 oz) black beans, drained and rinsed
- 1 cup corn kernels (fresh or frozen)
- 1 cup diced tomatoes (canned or fresh)
- 1 teaspoon ground cumin
- 1 teaspoon chili powder
- Salt and pepper, to taste
- Fresh cilantro or parsley (for garnish)

Instructions:

1. Preheat the oven. Preheat the oven to 375° Fahrenheit (190° Celsius). Prepare the bell peppers. Cut off the tops of the bell peppers and remove the seeds.

2. Lightly oil a baking dish and arrange the bell peppers inside. To cook quinoa, blend it with vegetable broth in a pot.

3. Bring to a boil, then reduce the heat and simmer for 15 minutes, or until the quinoa is cooked and the liquid has been absorbed.

4. Make the filling: In a large mixing bowl, combine the cooked quinoa, black beans, corn, diced tomatoes, ground cumin, chilli powder, salt and pepper.

5. Stuff the bell peppers. Fill the bell peppers with the quinoa mixture. Put the tops back on the peppers. To bake, cover the baking dish with foil.

6. Bake for thirty minutes. Remove the foil and bake for another 10 minutes. Serve and Enjoy! Garnish with fresh parsley or cilantro.

Nutritional Information (per serving):

Calories: Approximately 350 kcal

Protein: 12 g

Carbohydrates: 65 g

Fiber: 12 g

Fat: 5 g

Lentil Soup with Whole Wheat Crackers

Ingredients:

- 2 liters vegetable or ham stock
- 150g red lentils
- 6 carrots, finely chopped
- 2 medium leeks, sliced (about 300g)
- Small handful of chopped parsley, to serve

Instructions:

1. In a large pan, heat the stock and add the lentils. Bring to a boil, then let the lentils to soften for a few minutes.

2. Season with the carrots and leeks (if using gammon stock, do not add salt because it will make it excessively salty).

3. Bring to a boil, then reduce heat, cover, and simmer for 45 minutes to an hour,

or until the lentils have broken down. Sprinkle with parsley and serve with buttered bread, if desired.

Nutritional Information (per serving):

Calories: Approximately 219 kcal

Fat: 3 g

Saturates: 0.3 g

Carbohydrates: 33 g

Sugars: 11 g

Fiber: 9 g

Protein: 12 g

Salt: 1.4 g

Greek Yogurt Parfait with Berries and Almonds

Ingredients:

- 1 cup Greek yogurt (plain or vanilla)
- 1/2 cup mixed berries (such as strawberries, blueberries, and raspberries)
- 2 tablespoons sliced almonds
- 1 teaspoon honey (optional)

Instructions:

1. Layer the Parfait. In a glass, bowl, food container, or mason jar, layer the ingredients in this order:

2. Begin with a teaspoon of crushed cookies (optional). Spread a layer of Greek yoghurt.

3. Finish with a layer of mixed berries. Repeat the layers until you've reached the top of the container.

4. Finish with a sprinkling of chopped almonds.

5. Serve and Enjoy! Enjoy this delicious and healthful Greek Yoghurt Parfait with Berries and Almonds.

Nutritional Information (per serving):

Calories: Approximately 250 kcal

Protein: 15 g

Carbohydrates: 20 g

Fiber: 5 g

Fat: 6 g

05

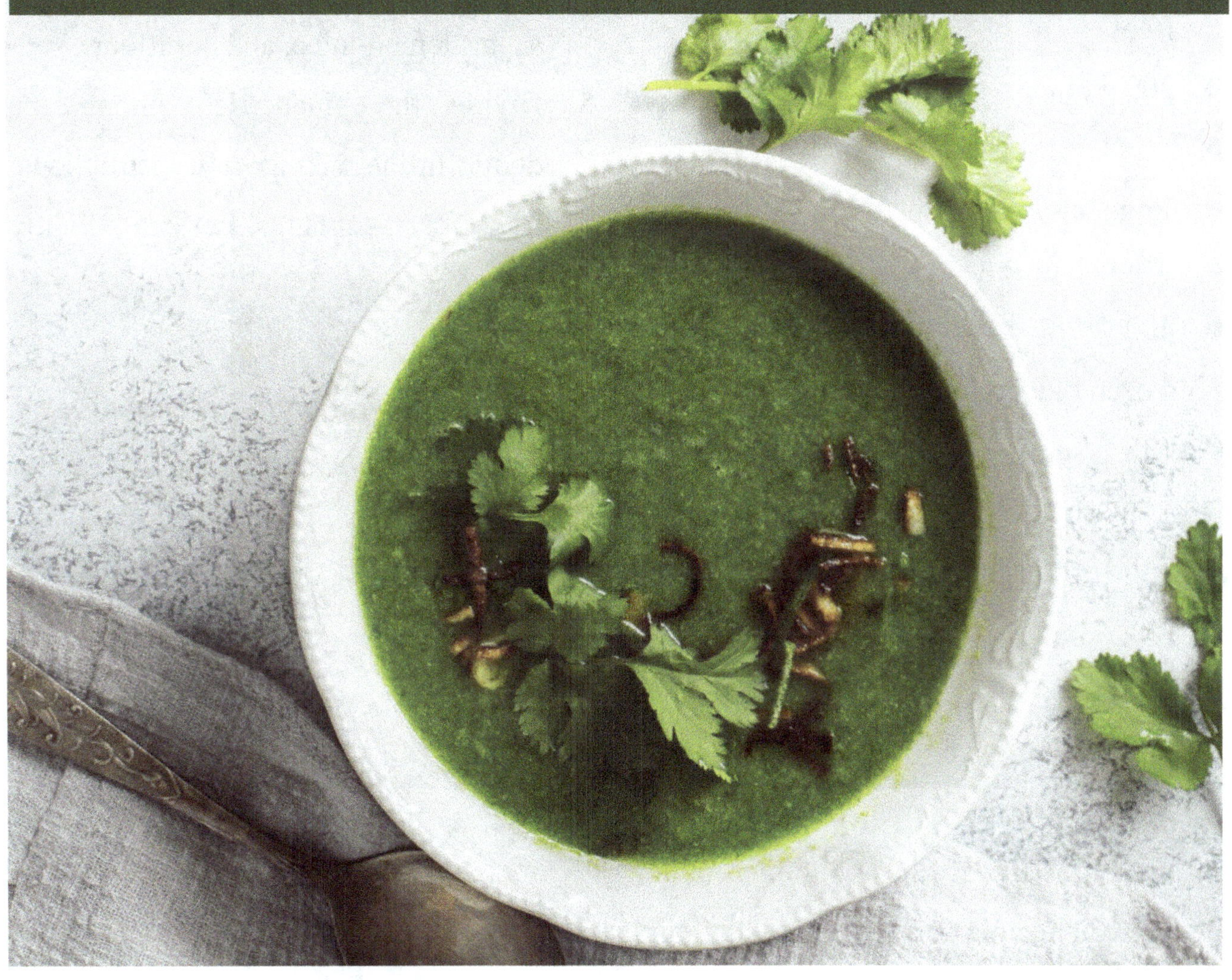

Ingredients:

- 350 – 400 g (2 1/2 cups – 3 cups) gluten-free flour (make sure the flour doesn't contain ingredients that are high in FODMAPs)
- 210 g (1 3/4 stick) cold butter (you can also replace this with lactose-free margarine to make the recipe lactose-free)
- 200 g (1 cup) sugar
- 5 g (1 + 1/4 tsp) baking powder
- 1 egg, at room temperature
- A pinch of salt
- 400 g (4 cups) blueberries (I used frozen blueberries that I defrosted first)
- 1 tbsp sugar
- 1 splash of lemon juice
- 1 tbsp cornstarch

Instructions:

1. Preheat the oven. Preheat the oven to 180 °C. Cut the butter into pieces and combine all of the bottom/crumble ingredients in a bowl. Knead with your hands until the dough is crumbly.

2. Make sure the butter is thoroughly blended into the dough mixture and that there are no huge lumps of butter in it.

3. Line a baking tin with baking parchment and spread half of the crumble mixture over the bottom. Press it into the bottom with your fingertips.

4. Combine the blueberries with the sugar, lemon juice, and cornflour.

5. Divide the blueberries among the dough in the baking tray. Instructions: Bake for 35 minutes. Let cool slightly before serving.

Nutritional Information (per serving):
Calories: Approximately 250 kcal
Protein: 2 g
Carbohydrates: 60 g
Fiber: 4 g
Fat: 10 g

Ingredients:

- 4 cups crispy rice cereal (such as Rice Krispies)
- 1/4 cup unsalted butter
- 1 package (10 oz) marshmallows
- 1 teaspoon pumpkin spice blend (or a mix of cinnamon, nutmeg, and allspice)
- 1/2 teaspoon vanilla extract
- Cooking spray or extra butter (for greasing the pan)

Instructions:

1. Prepare the pan: Coat a 9x9-inch baking pan with cooking spray or additional butter.
2. Melt butter and marshmallows: In a large saucepan, melt the butter over low heat. Add the marshmallows and whisk until melted and smooth.
3. Remove from heat. Stir in pumpkin spice (or cinnamon, nutmeg, allspice) and vanilla essence.
4. Mix with rice cereal. Combine the crispy rice cereal with the marshmallow mixture. Stir until thoroughly blended. Press into the pan.
5. Transfer the mixture to a prepared baking pan. Use a spatula or your hands to press it down evenly.
6. Allow goodies to cool for 30 minutes before cutting. Cut into squares or bars.
7. Serve and Enjoy! Enjoy these delicious Pumpkin Spice Rice Krispie Treats!

Nutritional Information (per serving):
Calories: Approximately 150 kcal
Carbohydrates: 30 g
Fat: 3 g
Protein: 1 g

Cantaloupe and Prosciutto Skewers

Ingredients:

- 1 ripe cantaloupe (about 350g/12oz), halved and seeded
- 8 thin slices of prosciutto
- Fresh basil leaves
- Balsamic glaze (optional, for drizzling)

Instructions:

1. Prepare the cantaloupe: Cut the cantaloupe into bite-sized chunks or use a melon baller to form little melon balls.

2. Wrap with prosciutto: Fold a slice of prosciutto in half lengthwise. Wrap each melon cube or ball in a slice of prosciutto. Thread them onto a thin skewer or toothpick.

3. Assemble the Skewers Place a fresh basil leaf between the melon and prosciutto on each skewer.

4. Serve and Enjoy! Drizzle with balsamic glaze if desired. Enjoy these delicious Cantaloupe and Prosciutto Skewers!

Nutritional Information (per serving):

Calories: Approximately 60 kcal

Protein: 3 g

Carbohydrates: 5 g

Fat: 3 g

Baked Cinnamon Banana Chips

Ingredients:

- 2 ripe bananas
- 1 tablespoon lemon juice
- 1 teaspoon coconut oil (optional)
- 1 teaspoon ground cinnamon

Instructions

1. Preheat the Oven: Start by setting your oven to 200°F (93°C) so it can warm up.

2. Slice the Bananas: Cut the bananas into thin, round slices, aiming for about 1/4 inch thick.

3. Toss with Lemon Juice: Mix the banana slices with lemon juice. This helps keep them from turning brown.

4. Arrange on a Baking Sheet: Line a baking sheet with parchment paper, then lay out the banana slices in a single layer.

5. Brush with Coconut Oil (Optional): If you like, you can lightly brush the banana slices with melted coconut oil to add some extra flavor.

6. Sprinkle with Cinnamon: Evenly sprinkle ground cinnamon over the banana slices.

7. Bake: Put the baking sheet in the oven and bake for 2-3 hours. The banana chips should become crispy and slightly browned around the edges. Keep an eye on them so they don't burn.

8. Cool and Enjoy: Once they're out of the oven, let the banana chips cool for a few minutes so they can harden.

Nutritional Information (per serving):

Calories: Approximately 73 kcal

Carbohydrates: 19 g

Fiber: 2 g

Fat: 0 g

Protein: 1 g

Greek Yogurt Parfait with Berries and Almonds

Ingredients:

- 1 cup Greek yogurt (plain or vanilla)
- 1/2 cup mixed berries (such as strawberries, blueberries, and raspberries)
- 2 tablespoons sliced almonds
- 1 teaspoon honey (optional)

Instructions:

1. Layer the Parfait. In a glass, bowl, food container, or mason jar, layer the ingredients in this order:

2. Begin with a teaspoon of crushed cookies (optional). Spread a layer of Greek yoghurt.

3. Finish with a layer of mixed berries. Repeat the layers until you've reached the top of the container.

4. Finish with a sprinkling of chopped almonds. Serve and Enjoy! Enjoy this delicious and healthful Greek Yoghurt Parfait with Berries and Almonds

Nutritional Information (per serving):

Calories: Approximately 250 kcal

Protein: 15 g

Carbohydrates: 20 g

Fiber: 5 g

Fat: 6 g

Chia Seed Pudding with Kiwi

Ingredients:

- 2/3 cup chia seeds
- 1 1/2 cups dairy-free milk of your choice (such as almond milk or oat milk)
- 1 1/4 tablespoons agave syrup (or sweetener of your preference)
- 1 teaspoon vanilla extract
- 4 kiwi fruits, peeled and diced
- 1/2 cup fresh blueberries
- 1 tablespoon toasted coconut flakes

Instructions:

1. Prepare the Chia Pudding: In a dish, combine the chia seeds, dairy-free milk, agave syrup, and vanilla essence.
2. Stir thoroughly to mix. Divide the mixture into tiny serving jars or containers. Cover and refrigerate for at least 1-2 hours, preferably overnight. Give them a brisk stir from time to time to ensure that the seeds absorb the majority of the liquid.
3. Create the Kiwi Topping: Puree the peeled kiwi fruits. Pour the kiwi puree on top of the chilled chia pudding.
4. Garnish and serve. Garnish with additional diced kiwi, fresh blueberries, and toasted coconut flakes.
5. Enjoy this delicious and healthful Chia Seed Pudding with Kiwi!

Nutritional Information (per serving):

Calories: Approximately 250 kcal

Protein: 15 g

Carbohydrates: 20 g

Fiber: 5 g

Fat: 6 g

Dark Chocolate-Dipped Strawberries

Ingredients:

- 3 ounces quality dark chocolate, chopped
- 12 large strawberries

Prep time	Calories
30 minute	43

Instructions:

1. Rinse the strawberries under cold water. If they're organic, a simple rinse in a strainer will do. For regular strawberries, soak them in a bowl with four parts water and one part white vinegar for 20 minutes, then rinse.

2. Microwave 2/3 of the chopped dark chocolate in a small bowl on medium for 1 minute. Stir and continue microwaving in 20-second bursts until fully melted, aiming for 110°F (43°C).

3. Put the remaining 1/3 of the dark chocolate in a piping bag or a small plastic sandwich bag, and snip off a tiny corner.

4. Hold each strawberry by the stem, dip it into the melted chocolate, and let the excess drip off. Place the dipped strawberries on a parchment-lined baking sheet.

5. Drizzle the melted chocolate over the strawberries using the piping bag, creating any patterns or designs you like.

6. Refrigerate the strawberries for 15-20 minutes until the chocolate sets

Rice Pudding with Cinnamon

Ingredients:

- 1 cup medium grain white rice (uncooked)
- 4 cups milk
- 1/2 cup sugar
- 1 teaspoon vanilla extract
- 1/2 cup sultanas (raisins)
- 1 cinnamon stick

Prep time	Calories
5 minutes	200 (1 cup serving)

Instructions:

1. Butter a casserole dish with a capacity of at least ten cups. In a saucepan over medium-high heat, combine the milk, sugar, and vanilla.
2. Bring to a simmer, stirring to dissolve the sugar, until the surface foams (don't boil or it will split). Place the rice, sultanas, and cinnamon stick in the prepared baking dish.
3. Pour the milk mixture over the rice and stir well. Cover the baking dish with either a lid or aluminium foil.
4. Bake at 325°F (160°C) for about 2 hours, until the rice is soft and the custard is thick and creamy. Before serving, make sure to remove the cinnamon stick.

Low FODMAP Trail Mix

Ingredients:

- 50g mixed unsalted nuts (e.g., almonds, walnuts, or macadamia nuts), chopped
- 60g pumpkin seeds
- 60g sunflower seeds
- 130g dried cranberries
- 30g dark chocolate chips (omit if the trail mix will be exposed to heat)
- 30g unsweetened coconut flakes or toasted coconut chips (omit if needing refined sugar-free)
- 30g rolled oats (optional; omit if you prefer a grain-free trail mix)
- Pinch of sea salt

Prep time	Calories
5 minutes	200 calories per serving.

Instructions:

1. In a large mixing bowl, combine mixed nuts, pumpkin seeds, sunflower seeds, dried cranberries, dark chocolate chips, oats (optional), and coconut flakes or toasted coconut chips.

2. Add a pinch of sea salt to the dry ingredients. Gently toss and combine all of the ingredients until evenly distributed.

3. Keep your low FODMAP trail mix in an airtight container or zip-top bag.

Nutritional Information (per serving, approximately ½ cup):

Calories: Approximately 200 calories per serving.

Baked Apple Slices with Cinnamon

Ingredients:

- 4 medium-sized apples (such as Granny Smiths, Honeycrisps, or Fujis)
- 2 tablespoons unsalted butter, melted
- 2 tablespoons light brown sugar
- 1 teaspoon ground cinnamon
- 1/4 teaspoon ground nutmeg
- 1/2 teaspoon vanilla extract
- Pinch of salt

Prep time	calories
10 minutes	100

Instructions:

1. Preheat the oven to 350°F (175° C). Line a baking sheet with parchment paper. Peel, core, and cut apples into thin rounds. In a large mixing basin, add melted butter, brown sugar, cinnamon, nutmeg, vanilla essence, and a pinch of salt.

2. Toss the apple slices in the bowl until uniformly covered with butter and seasonings. Arrange the coated apple slices in a single layer on the prepared baking sheet, taking care not to overlap them. Bake for 20 to 25 minutes, or until the apples are soft and begin to caramelise.

3. Warm baked apple slices can be served on their own or with whipped cream or vanilla ice cream.

Nutritional Information (per serving):

Calories: Approximately 100 calories per serving (based on 1 medium apple).

06

Green Salad with Chopped Vegetables and Avocado

Ingredients:

- 4 cups mixed salad greens
- 1 ripe avocado, sliced
- 1 cucumber, sliced
- 1 cup cherry tomatoes, halved
- 1/4 red onion, thinly sliced
- 1/4 cup feta cheese, crumbled
- 1/4 cup toasted pine nuts

Prep time
10 minute

Instructions:

1. In a large salad bowl, toss together the mixed salad greens, avocado, cucumber, cherry tomatoes, red onion, crumbled feta cheese, and toasted pine nuts.

2. To ensure thorough mixing, lightly toss the components. You may either use your favourite store-bought dressing or make your own vinaigrette with olive oil, lemon juice, salt, and pepper.

3. Pour the dressing over the salad and toss to evenly coat the contents.

4. Serve the Green Salad with Avocado immediately and enjoy!

Quinoa and Chickpea Salad

Ingredients:

- 1 cup quinoa
- 2 cups water
- 1 (15-ounce) can chickpeas (garbanzo beans), drained and rinsed
- 1 large cucumber, diced
- 1 red bell pepper, diced
- 1 cup cherry tomatoes, halved
- 1/4 red onion, finely chopped
- 1/2 cup fresh parsley, chopped
- 1/4 cup fresh mint leaves, chopped
- 1/2 cup crumbled feta cheese (optional)
- Salt and pepper, to taste

Dressing:

- 3 tablespoons extra-virgin olive oil
- Juice of 1 lemon
- 1 garlic clove, minced
- 1 teaspoon dried oregano
- Salt and pepper, to taste

Prep time	Calories
15 minutes	363

Instructions:

1. Rinse the quinoa with cool water. In a medium saucepan, mix together the quinoa and water.

2. Bring to a boil, then reduce heat and simmer for 15 minutes, or until the quinoa is cooked and the water has been absorbed.

3. Fluff with a fork and allow to cool. In a large salad bowl, mix together the cooked quinoa, chickpeas, cucumber, red bell pepper, cherry tomatoes, red onion, parsley, and mint.

4. To create the dressing, combine olive oil, lemon juice, minced garlic, dried oregano, salt, and pepper in a small mixing dish.

5. Pour the dressing over the salad and mix until thoroughly incorporated. If using, put crumbled feta cheese over top. Season with more salt and pepper if necessary. Serve chilled or room temperature.

Nutritional Information (per serving):

Calories: Approximately 363 calories per serving.

Roasted Beet Salad with Feta

Ingredients:

- 4 beets, trimmed, leaving 1 inch of stems attached
- ¼ cup minced shallot
- 2 tablespoons minced fresh parsley
- 2 tablespoons extra-virgin olive oil
- 1 tablespoon balsamic vinegar
- Salt and pepper, to taste
- ¼ cup crumbled feta cheese
- Prep Time: Approximately 15 minutes (plus roasting time for beets)

Instructions:

1. Preheat the oven to 400 °F (200 °C). Wrap each beetroot individually in aluminium foil and lay on a baking sheet. Roast the beets in a preheated oven until easily pierced with a fork (approximately 45 minutes to an hour).

2. Let the roasted beets cool until you can handle them. Peel the beets and cut into 1/4-inch slices. While the beets roast, prepare the vinaigrette by

whisking together the minced shallots, fresh parsley, olive oil, balsamic vinegar, salt, and pepper in a bowl.

3. Place the warm sliced beets on a serving platter. Pour the vinaigrette over the beets and top with crumbled feta.

Nutritional Information (per serving):

Calories: Approximately 149 calories per serving.

Cabbage Slaw with Carrots and Apple

Ingredients:

- 1/2 small red cabbage (about 3 cups), thinly sliced
- 2 cups shredded carrots
- 1 red apple, chopped (you can slice it thin or cut into cubes)
- 1/2 cup fresh parsley, chopped (optional, adjust to taste)
- 1/4 red onion, thinly sliced
- 1/4 cup pumpkin seeds (raw or roasted)

Dressing:

- 1/2 cup mayonnaise (use a non-dairy version if preferred)
- 1 tablespoon apple cider vinegar
- Salt, to taste

Prep time	Calories
15 minutes	149

Instructions:

1. Shred the carrots with a cheese grater, food processor, or mandolin slicer. Slice the red cabbage into thin strips. Cut the apples into thin slices or small cubes.

2. In a large serving bowl, mix together the cabbage, carrots, apple, red onion, parsley, and pumpkin seeds.

3. To prepare the dressing, mix together the mayonnaise, apple cider vinegar, and salt in a small bowl.

4. Pour the dressing over the salad and toss until evenly coated. Serve and enjoy this cool Cabbage Slaw with Carrots and Apple!

Nutritional Information (per serving):

Calories: Approximately 149 calories per serving.

Spinach and Strawberry Salad

Ingredients:

- Fresh Spinach: 4 cups, washed and dried
- Strawberries: 2 cups, hulled and sliced
- Almonds: 1/2 cup, sliced or slivered, toasted
- Poppy Seed Dressing:
- Olive oil: 1/4 cup
- White wine vinegar: 2 tablespoons
- Honey: 2 tablespoons
- Dijon mustard: 1 tablespoon
- Poppy seeds: 1 teaspoon
- Salt and pepper to taste

Prep time	Calories
10 minutes	149

Instructions:

1. To prepare, whisk together olive oil, white wine vinegar, honey, Dijon mustard, and poppy seeds in a small bowl.
2. Add salt and pepper to taste, and balance the sweetness and acidity to your liking.
3. Salad Assembly: In a large bowl, combine fresh spinach and cut strawberries. Drizzle the dressing over the salad and gently toss to distribute evenly.
4. Sprinkle roasted almonds on top for a delicious crunch. Serve immediately to really appreciate the fresh spinach, luscious strawberries, and crisp almonds.

Nutritional Information (per serving):
Calories: Approximately 149 calories per serving.

Greek Salad with Quinoa

Ingredients:

- 1 cup quinoa
- 1 1/2 cups water
- 1 cucumber, diced
- 1/2 red onion, finely chopped
- 1 cup grape tomatoes, halved
- 1/2 cup Kalamata olives, pitted and sliced
- 1 (15-ounce) can chickpeas (garbanzo beans), drained and rinsed
- 1/2 cup crumbled feta cheese (optional; omit for a vegan version)
- Fresh parsley or mint leaves for garnish

Dressing:

- 2 cloves garlic, minced
- 1 teaspoon dried oregano
- Juice of 1 lemon
- 2 tablespoons red wine vinegar
- 1/4 cup extra-virgin olive oil
- Salt and pepper, to taste
- Prep Time: Approximately 15 minutes (plus cooking time for quinoa)

Instructions:

1. Wash the quinoa in cold water through a fine mesh strainer. Stir together the water, a little salt, and rinsed quinoa in a medium saucepan. Over medium heat, bring to a boil; then, lower to a simmer and cook, stirring, until the water is absorbed, about 15 minutes.

2. The finished quinoa should have a tiny white ring around each piece. After taking the quinoa off of the stove, give it a fork fluff and let it come to room temperature.

3. Combine the chilled quinoa, chopped red onion, halved grape tomatoes, sliced Kalamata olives, and chickpeas in a big bowl.

4. Top with crumbled feta cheese, if desired. Whisk together the extra-virgin olive oil, lemon juice, red wine vinegar, dried oregano, and minced garlic for the dressing.

5. Spoon the dressing over the salad and thoroughly mix everything. Top with mint or parsley leaves. Give cold or room temperature service.

Nutritional Information (per serving):

Calories: Approximately 500 calories per serving.

Mixed Bean Salad

Ingredients:

- 1 x 400g tin mixed bean salad, drained and rinsed
- 2 spring onions, finely chopped
- 2 celery sticks, thinly sliced
- 1 large tomato, deseeded and finely diced

Dressing:

- 3 tbsp olive oil
- 1 tbsp white wine vinegar
- 1 tsp sugar
- 2 tsp Dijon mustard
- 1 tbsp chopped fresh tarragon
- 1 tbsp chopped fresh parsley

Instructions:

1. Put all the salad ingredients in a bowl and thoroughly combine.
2. Thoroughly combine the dressing ingredients in a different basin or bottle. Toss together, then drizzle dressing over salad and season with salt and pepper.
3. The flavours will meld over the course of two to three days in the refrigerator, covered.

Watermelon and Mint Salad

Ingredients:

- 4 cups diced watermelon
- 1 cup crumbled feta cheese
- 1/4 cup fresh mint leaves, chopped
- Zest of 1 lemon
- Juice of 1 lemon
- 2 tablespoons extra-virgin olive oil

Instructions:

1. Gather the chopped mint leaves, crumbled feta cheese, and cubed watermelon in a big basin.
2. Whisk the olive oil, lemon juice, and zest together in a small dish. Spoon the dressing over the watermelon mixture and toss just enough to incorporate.
3. Present straight away and savour this cool salad!

Nutrition Facts (per serving):

Calories: Approximately 56 calories per 3/4-cup serving

Broccoli and Cranberry Salad

Ingredients:

- 2 cups broccoli florets
- 1/4 cup dried cranberries (unsweetened)
- 1/4 cup slivered almonds
- 1/4 cup plain Greek yogurt
- 1 tablespoon honey
- 1 tablespoon apple cider vinegar
- Salt to taste

Prep time	Kilocalories per serving
15 minutes	150

Instructions:

1. Get the Broccoli Ready: Trim the broccoli to little, bite-sized florets. Toss in the dressing. Add the apple cider vinegar, honey, and Greek yoghurt to a small bowl. Give it a good swirl.

2. Combine ingredients: To a big bowl, add the slivered almonds, dried cranberries, and broccoli florets.

3. Dress First: Dollop the broccoli mixture with the dressing. Once the broccoli is well coated, toss everything together.

4. Winter: Season with a little salt. Deliver: For a fresher flavour, the salad can be served right away or refrigerated for an hour.

Avocado and Tomato Salad

Ingredients:

- 1 ripe avocado, diced
- 2 medium tomatoes, diced
- 1 small cucumber, peeled and diced
- 1/4 red onion, finely chopped (optional)
- 1 tablespoon olive oil
- 1 tablespoon lemon juice
- Salt and pepper to taste
- Fresh basil leaves for garnish (optional)

Prep time	Kilocalories
10 minutes	200

Instructions:

1. Start the Vegetables: Halve the tomatoes and avocado. Peel and chop the cucumber. If used, finely cut the red onion.

2. Toss the salad: To a big bowl, add the diced red onion, cucumber, tomatoes, and avocado.

3. Deck the Salad: Pour over the salad the lemon juice and olive oil. Turn the vegetables over gently to coat them all.

4. Winter: Tailor with salt and pepper. Deliver: Should you so choose, garnish with fresh basil leaves. Deliver right away.

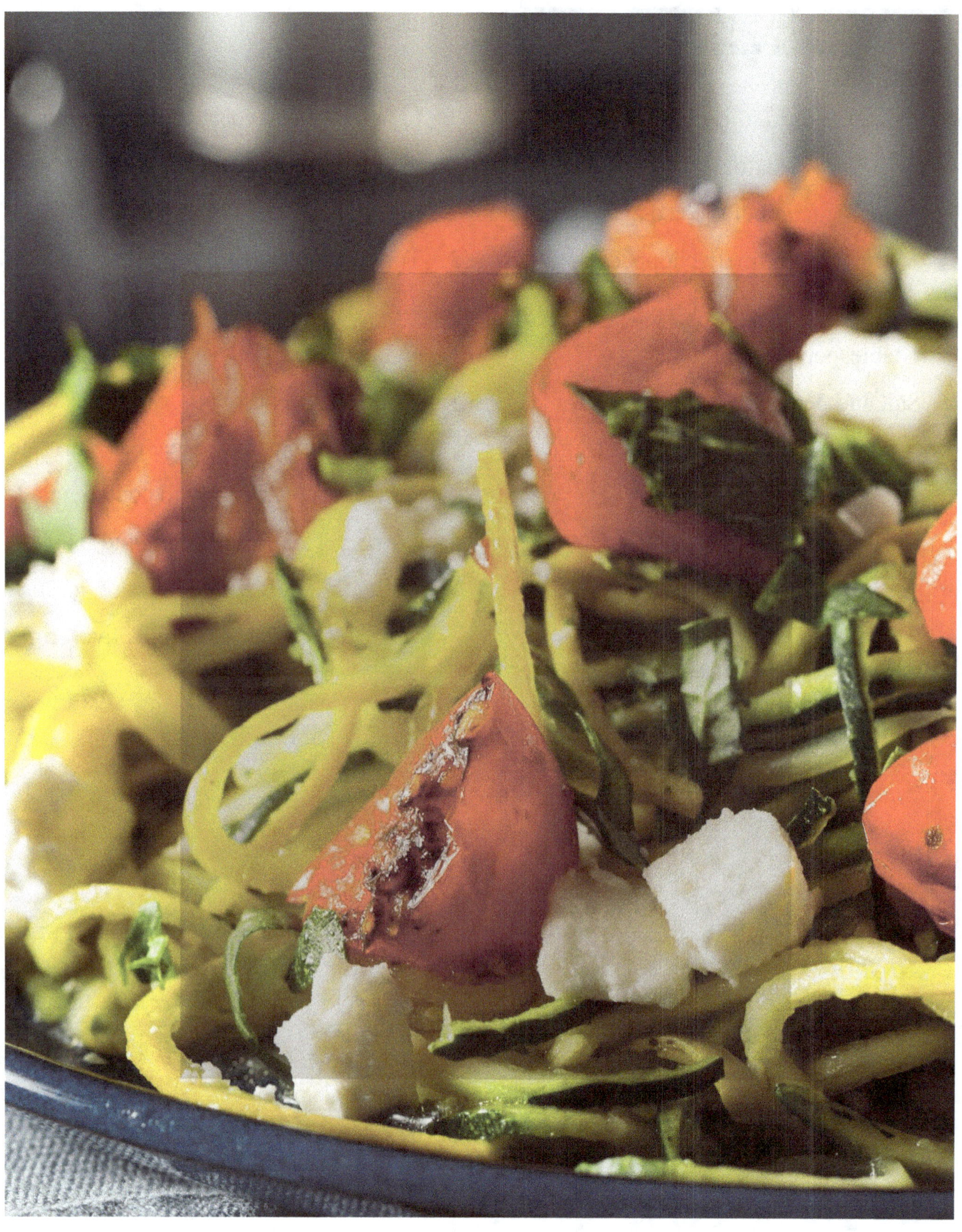

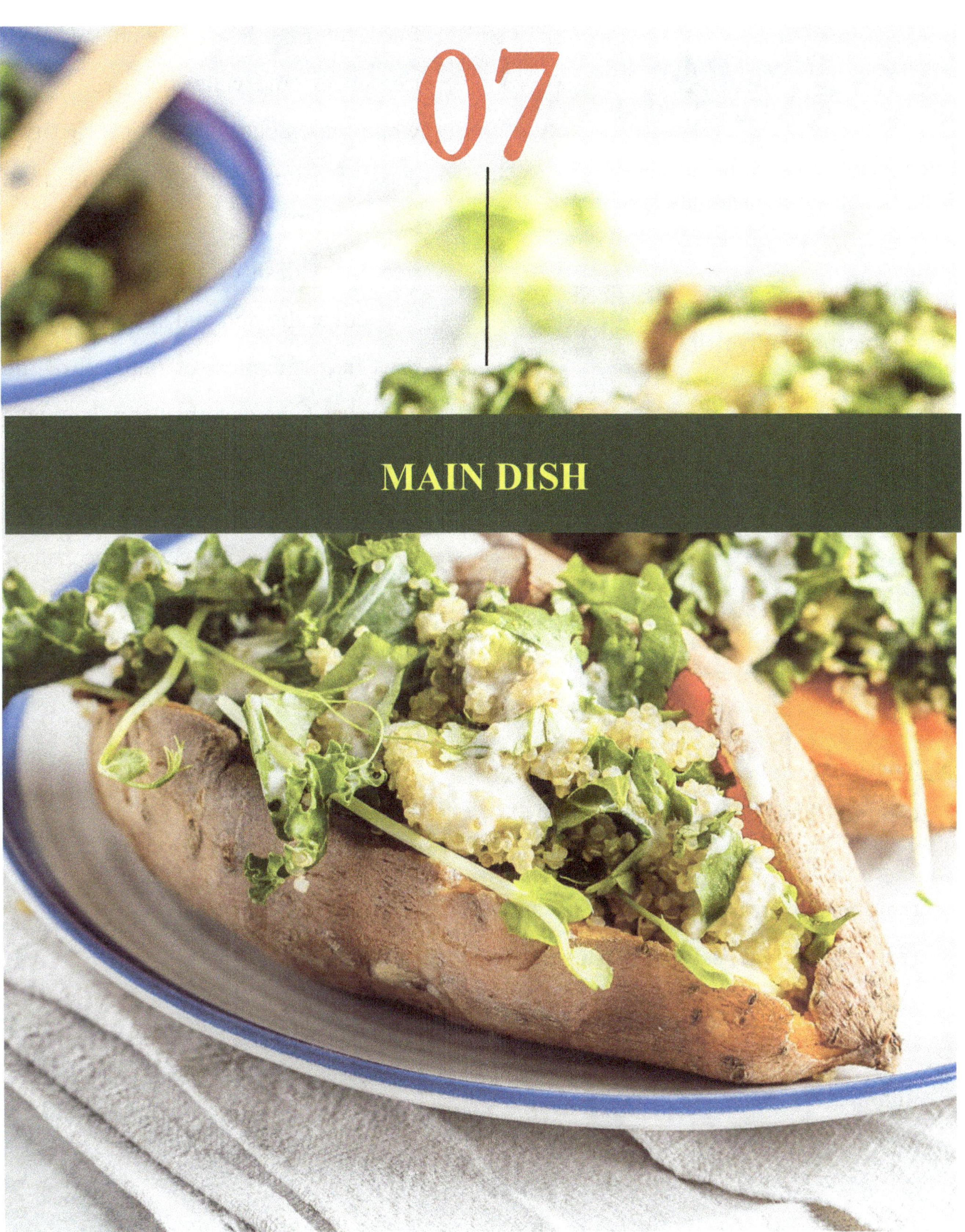

07

MAIN DISH

Ingredients:

- 2 boneless, skinless chicken breasts
- 1 cup white rice
- 2 large carrots, peeled and sliced
- 1 tablespoon olive oil
- Salt (to taste)
- Pepper (to taste, optional)
- 2 cups water

Prep time	Kilocalories
30 minutes	350kcal

Instructions:

1. Get the Chicken Ready: Heat your grill or grill pan over medium-high. Drizzle the chicken breasts with olive oil and season just with salt (and pepper, if you'd want).

2. Grill the chicken for six to seven minutes on each side, or until the internal temperature reaches 165°F (75°C).

3. Cook the rice. Rinse one cup of white rice under cold water till it runs clean while the chicken is roasting. Get two cups of water to a boil in a medium saucepan. To the boiling water add the rice and a dash of salt. Turn down to low, cover the pot, and simmer the rice for fifteen minutes, or until all of the water has been absorbed and the rice is soft. Cook the carrots in steam.

4. As the rice cooks, set the sliced carrots in a steamer basket over a saucepan of boiling water. Steam the carrots, covered, for five to seven minutes, or until they are soft but not mush.

5. Serving: Divide the cooked rice, steaming carrots, and grilled chicken between two plates when everything is done. Savour your dinner!

Baked Cod with Mashed Potatoes and Green Beans

Ingredients:

For the Cod:

- 4 cod fillets (about 150g each)
- 2 tablespoons olive oil
- 1 lemon (sliced)
- 1 teaspoon dried oregano
- Salt and pepper to taste

For the Mashed Potatoes:

- 4 medium potatoes (peeled and cubed)
- 2 tablespoons butter
- 1/4 cup milk (or as needed)
- Salt to taste

For the Green Beans:

- 400g green beans (trimmed)
- 1 tablespoon olive oil
- Salt and pepper to taste

Prep time	Kilocalories	Cooking
15 minutes	400	25 minutes

Instructions:

1. Preheat the oven: Preheat the oven to 200°C (400°F). Prepare the cod. Place the cod fillets onto a baking sheet. Drizzle with olive oil and season with oregano, salt and pepper. Lay lemon wedges on top of each fillet.

2. Bake the fish for 15-20 minutes, or until it is opaque and readily flaked with a fork.

3. Cook the potatoes. While the cod bakes, cook the cubed potatoes in a large saucepan of water for 10-15 minutes, or until soft.

4. Drain the potatoes and return to the pot. Add the butter and milk, then mash until smooth. If necessary, increase the amount of milk. Add salt to taste.

5. Prepare the Green Beans: Bring water to a boil in a big pot, then add green beans. Cook for 5-7 minutes, until tender yet still crisp. Drain the beans and stir them with olive oil, salt, and pepper.

6. Serve: Serve the baked fish fillets with mashed potatoes and green beans as a side. Have a great meal!

Scrambled Eggs with Toast and Fruit Juice

Ingredients

- 2 large eggs
- 1 tablespoon water
- 1 teaspoon olive oil or a small pat of butter
- 1 slice of white or whole-wheat bread
- 1 cup of diluted fruit juice (like apple or grape juice)
- Salt (optional, in small amounts)
- Pepper (optional, in small amounts)

Prep time	Kilocalories
10 minutes	250

Instructions:

1. Prepare the eggs: Break the eggs into a basin. Add one tablespoon of water. Use a fork to thoroughly combine the eggs.

2. Cook the eggs: Preheat a nonstick pan over medium heat. Pour 1 teaspoon olive oil or a little pat of butter into the pan. Pour the beaten eggs into the pan. Stir gently with a spatula until the eggs are softly scrambled and fully cooked. This should take approximately 3-5 minutes. Toast the bread. While the eggs cook, toast a slice of bread in the toaster.

3. Prepare the juice: Pour 1 cup of apple or grape juice into a glass. If the juice is excessively powerful, dilute it with the same amount of water.

4. Serve: Put the scrambled eggs on a platter. Add the toast to the platter. Serve with a glass of diluted fruit juice.

Tomato Soup with Crackers and a Grilled Cheese Sandwich

Tomato Soup:

- 4 cups low-sodium vegetable broth
- 1 can (28 oz) low-sodium crushed tomatoes
- 1 medium carrot, peeled and chopped
- 1 celery stalk, chopped
- 1 small onion, chopped
- 1 clove garlic, minced
- 1 tablespoon olive oil
- 1 teaspoon dried basil
- 1 teaspoon dried oregano
- Salt and pepper to taste

Crackers:

- Low-fiber, low-fat crackers (check label for diverticulitis-friendly options)

Grilled Cheese Sandwich:

- 2 slices white bread
- 1 slice low-fat cheese
- 1 teaspoon olive oil or butter

Prep time	Kilocalories
30 minutes	

Kilocalories per Serving:

Tomato Soup: 150 kcal

Crackers: 50 kcal (depending on the brand)

Grilled Cheese Sandwich: 250 kcal

Instructions:

1. Tomato Soup: Heat Oil: In a large pot, heat 1 tablespoon olive oil over medium heat. Cook the vegetables: Add the diced onion, carrot, and celery.
2. Cook for approximately 5 minutes, or until they begin to soften. Stir in the minced garlic and heat for a further minute. Ingredients: Combine the low-sodium vegetable broth, crushed tomatoes, dry basil, and dried oregano.
3. Stir to mix. Simmer: Bring the soup to a mild boil, then reduce heat and simmer for 15-20 minutes, or until the veggies are very soft.
4. Blend: Puree the soup with an immersion blender until smooth. (Alternatively, let it cool somewhat before blending in batches with a normal blender.)
5. Seasoning: Add salt and pepper to taste. Ladle the soup into individual bowls.

Cracker:

6. Serve low-fiber, low-fat crackers with soup. Grilled cheese sandwiches:
7. Prepare bread: Take two white pieces of bread. Place one piece of low-fat cheese between them.
8. Heat pan: Place a nonstick skillet over medium heat. Add one teaspoon of olive oil or butter.
9. Cook Sandwich: Place the sandwich in a skillet. Cook for 3-4 minutes on each side, or until the bread is golden brown

and the cheese has melted. Cut the sandwich in half and serve alongside the soup.

Turkey Meatballs with Zucchini Noodles

Ingredients:

For the Turkey Meatballs:

- 1 lb ground turkey
- 1 egg
- 1/2 cup rolled oats (blended into a coarse flour)
- 1/4 cup grated Parmesan cheese
- 1/2 teaspoon garlic powder
- 1/2 teaspoon onion powder
- 1/2 teaspoon dried oregano
- 1/2 teaspoon salt
- 1/4 teaspoon black pepper

For the Zucchini Noodles:

- 4 medium zucchinis (spiralized into noodles)
- 1 tablespoon olive oil
- 1/2 teaspoon garlic powder
- 1/4 teaspoon salt

Prep Time: Prep: 20 minutes

Cook: 20 minutes

Total: 40 minutes

Kilocalories per Serving: Approximately 300 kcal per serving

Instructions:

1. Preheat oven to 400 degrees Fahrenheit (200 degrees Celsius).
2. Prepare meatballs: In a large mixing bowl, add ground turkey, egg, oat flour, Parmesan cheese, garlic powder, onion powder, dried oregano, salt, and black pepper. Mix vigorously until all components are fully incorporated. Roll the mixture into small meatballs approximately an inch in diameter and place on a baking sheet lined with parchment paper.
3. Bake Meatballs: Place the baking sheet in a preheated oven. Bake for 18-20 minutes, or until the meatballs are thoroughly cooked and gently browned.
4. Cook Zucchini Noodles: While the meatballs bake, warm the olive oil in a large skillet over medium heat. Add the spiralized zucchini noodles to the skillet. Sprinkle with garlic powder and salt, then sauté for 3-5 minutes, or

until the noodles are soft but not mushy.

5. Serve: Divide the zucchini noodles among plates. Top with turkey meatballs. Enjoy your nutritious, diverticulitis-friendly lunch!

Greek Yogurt Tuna Salad Wraps

Ingredients:

- 1 can (5 oz) tuna, drained
- 1/2 cup plain Greek yogurt
- 1/4 cup finely chopped cucumber
- 1/4 cup finely chopped celery (optional)
- 1 tablespoon lemon juice
- 1 tablespoon fresh dill, chopped (or 1 teaspoon dried dill)
- Salt and pepper to taste
- 4 large lettuce leaves or whole-grain wraps

Prep time	Kilocalories
10 minutes	150

Instructions:

1. Prepare the tuna mixture: In a medium bowl, combine the drained tuna and Greek yoghurt.
2. Combine the finely diced cucumber, celery (if using), lemon juice, and dill.
3. Mix everything until well blended. Season with salt and pepper to taste.
4. Assemble the Wraps Spread out the lettuce leaves or whole-grain wrappers. Spoon the tuna mixture equally over each leaf or wrap.
5. If using lettuce, fold the edges over the filling and roll up. If using wraps, roll them securely. Serve: Serve immediately or refrigerate until later.

Sweet Potato and Chickpea Curry

Ingredients:

- 2 medium sweet potatoes, peeled and diced
- 1 can (15 oz) chickpeas, drained and rinsed
- 1 can (14 oz) diced tomatoes
- 1 cup low-sodium vegetable broth
- 1 small onion, finely chopped
- 2 cloves garlic, minced
- 1 tablespoon olive oil
- 1 teaspoon ground turmeric
- 1 teaspoon ground cumin
- 1 teaspoon ground coriander
- 1/2 teaspoon ground cinnamon
- 1/2 teaspoon ground ginger
- Salt and pepper to taste
- Fresh cilantro for garnish (optional)

Prep Time: 15 minutes prep

Cooking: 30 minutes

Total: 45 minutes

Kilocalories per Serving: Approximately 250 kcal per serving

Instructions:

1. Prepare the ingredients. Peel and dice the sweet potatoes. Finely cut the onion. Mince the garlic.

2. Cook the onions and garlic: In a large pot, warm the olive oil over medium heat. Add the chopped onion and simmer for 5 minutes, or until tender. Add the minced garlic and simmer for another minute.

3. Add the spices. Combine the ground turmeric, cumin, coriander, cinnamon, and ginger. Cook for 1-2 minutes, until the spices are fragrant. Add sweet potatoes and liquids. Add the diced sweet potatoes to the saucepan.

4. Pour in the diced tomatoes (with juice) and veggie broth. Stir to mix. Simmer the curry. Bring the mixture to a boil, then turn the heat down to low.

5. Cover the pot and boil for 20 minutes, or until the sweet potatoes are cooked.

6. Add chickpeas: Stir in the drained and rinsed chickpeas. Cook for a another 5-10 minutes, until well heated. Season and serve. Season with salt and

pepper to taste. Serve the curry hot, topped with fresh cilantro if preferred.

Baked Eggplant Parmesan

Ingredients:

- 1 large eggplant, sliced into 1/4-inch thick rounds
- 1 cup whole wheat breadcrumbs (or gluten-free breadcrumbs if needed)
- 1/2 cup grated Parmesan cheese
- 1 teaspoon dried oregano
- 1 teaspoon dried basil
- 2 large eggs, beaten
- 2 cups low-sodium marinara sauce
- 1 cup shredded part-skim mozzarella cheese
- Olive oil spray

Prep Time: 20 minutes

Cooking: 30 minutes

Kilocalories per Serving: Approximately 250 kcal

Instructions:

1. Preheat the oven. Preheat your oven to 375°F (190° C). Prepare the aubergine: Lightly spray both sides of the aubergine slices with olive oil. Arrange the slices on a baking sheet.

2. Bake the aubergine: Bake for 20 minutes in a preheated oven, flipping halfway through, until soft and faintly brown.

3. Bread the aubergine. In a bowl, combine the breadcrumbs, Parmesan cheese, oregano, and basil. Dip each eggplant slice in the beaten eggs and then coat with the breadcrumb mixture.

4. Layer the aubergine: In a baking dish, put a thin layer of marinara. Add a layer of breaded aubergine slices on top. Spoon extra marinara sauce over the aubergine, then top with mozzarella cheese.

5. Repeat the layers until all of the ingredients are utilised, ending with a layer of marinara sauce and mozzarella cheese.

6. Bake again. Bake for 10-15 minutes, or until the cheese melts and bubbles. Serve: Allow it cool for a few minutes before serving.

Quinoa-Stuffed Bell Peppers

Ingredients:

- 4 large bell peppers (any color)
- 1 cup quinoa
- 2 cups low-sodium vegetable broth
- 1 tablespoon olive oil
- 1 small onion, finely chopped
- 2 cloves garlic, minced
- 1 small zucchini, diced
- 1 carrot, grated
- 1 can (15 oz) diced tomatoes, drained
- 1 teaspoon dried oregano
- 1 teaspoon dried basil
- Salt and pepper to taste

Prep Time: 20 minutes preparation

Cooking: 30 minutes

Total: 50 minutes

Kilocalories per Serving: Approximately 200 kcal per stuffed pepper

Instructions:

1. Preheat and Prepare the Peppers: Preheat the oven to 375°F (190° C). Cut the bell pepper tops off and remove the seeds and membranes. Set aside.

2. Cook Quinoa: Rinse the quinoa with cool water. In a medium saucepan, heat the vegetable broth to a boil. Add the quinoa, decrease the heat to low, cover, and cook for about 15 minutes, or until cooked and the liquid is absorbed. Fluff with a fork, then set aside. Prepare the filling.

3. In a large skillet, heat the olive oil over medium heat. Add the diced zucchini and carrots. Sauté for about 5 minutes, until they begin to soften. Stir in the chopped spinach, drained tomatoes, oregano, basil, salt, and pepper. Cook for an additional 3-4 minutes, until the spinach has wilted.

4. Combine and Stuff: Combine the cooked quinoa and veggie combination. Stir well to combine. Spoon the quinoa-vegetable mixture into each bell pepper until it is full. Bake: Arrange the stuffed peppers vertically in a baking dish. Cover with foil and bake for 25-30 minutes or until the peppers are cooked. Serve: Allow to cool slightly before serving.

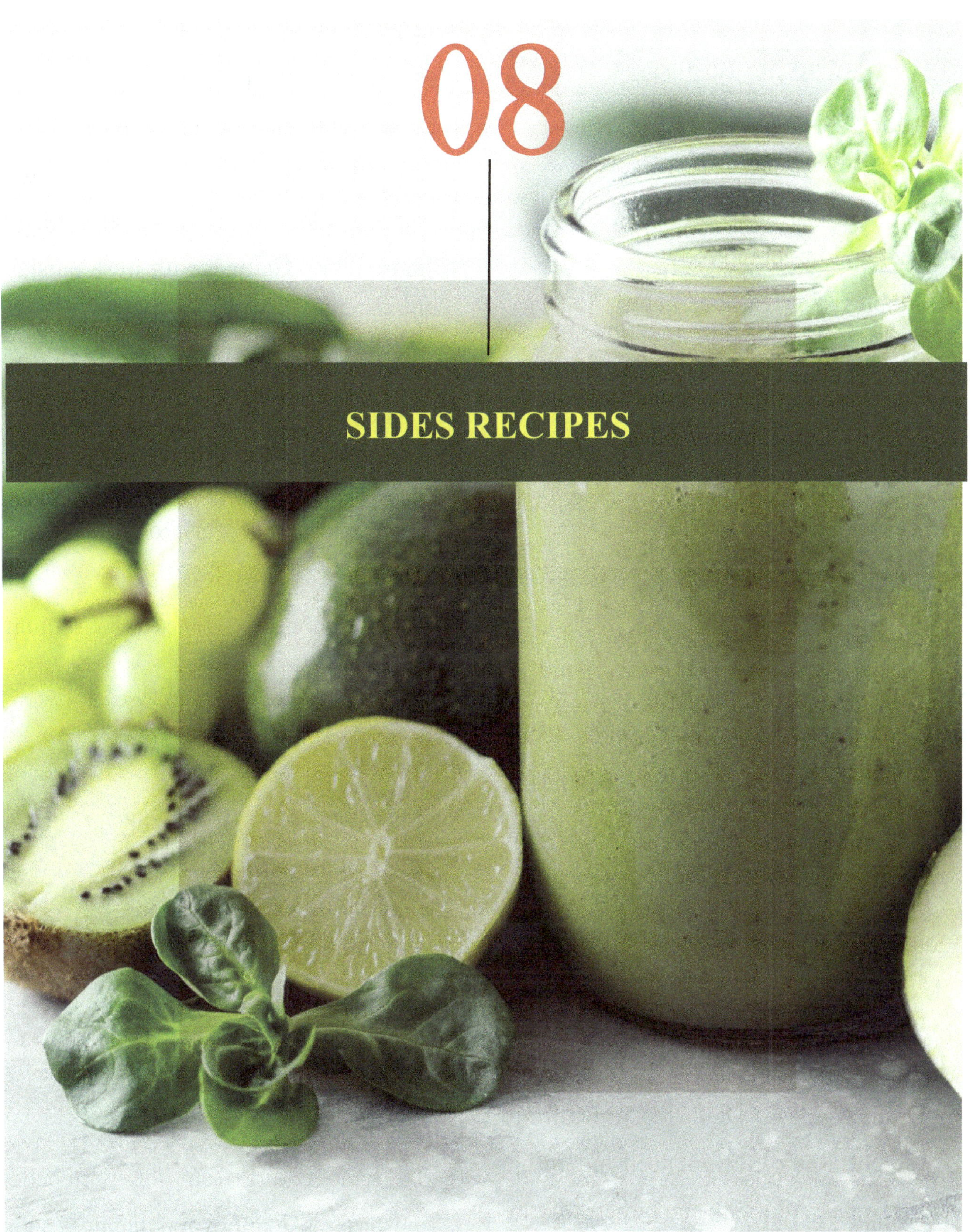

08
SIDES RECIPES

Garlic Mashed Potatoes

Ingredients:

- 4 large russet potatoes
- 3 cloves garlic
- 1/2 cup low-fat milk
- 2 tablespoons unsalted butter
- Salt to taste
- Fresh parsley (optional, for garnish)

Prep time	Kilocalories	Cook
10 minutes	200 kcal	20 minute

Instructions:

1. Peel and chop potatoes. Peel four big russet potatoes. Cut them into equal-sized bits for even cooking. Boil potatoes and garlic. Place the potato chunks and three peeled garlic cloves in a big pot. Cover with water and a dash of salt.

2. Bring to a boil over high heat, then reduce to medium and cook for 15-20 minutes, or until potatoes are cooked.

3. Drain & Mash: Drain the water from the pot. Return the potatoes and garlic to the pot. Add milk and butter. Mix in 1/2 cup low-fat milk and 2 tablespoons unsalted butter to the potatoes.

4. Mash until smooth. You can use either a potato masher or a fork. Season and serve. Add salt to taste and blend thoroughly. Garnish with fresh parsley for added colour. Serve warm.

Ginger-Marinated Grilled Portobello Mushrooms

Ingredients:

- 4 large portobello mushrooms
- 2 tablespoons olive oil
- 2 tablespoons soy sauce (low-sodium if possible)
- 2 tablespoons balsamic vinegar
- 2 cloves garlic, minced
- 1 teaspoon grated fresh ginger
- Salt and pepper to taste

Prep time	Kilocalories per servings
15 minute	120

Instructions:

1. To remove dirt from the portobello mushrooms, gently wipe them off with a moist cloth or paper towel. If the

stems are too tough, remove them. In a small bowl, combine the olive oil, soy sauce, balsamic vinegar, chopped garlic, and grated ginger.

2. Place the portobello mushrooms in a shallow dish and pour the marinade over them, coating both sides. Allow the mushrooms to marinade for approximately 10 minutes, flipping halfway through to ensure even flavour.

3. Preheat the grill to medium heat. If using a stovetop grill pan, preheat it to medium-high heat. Once the grill is hot, put the marinated mushrooms, gill side down. Grill for 4-5 minutes per side, or until tender and with grill marks. Season with salt and pepper to taste before serving.

4. Enjoy these delicious Ginger-Marinated Grilled Portobello Mushrooms as a healthful and diverticulitis-friendly lunch.

Ingredients:

- 1 pound carrots, peeled and sliced into rounds
- 2 tablespoons honey
- 1 tablespoon olive oil
- 1/4 teaspoon ground cinnamon
- Pinch of salt

Prep time	Kilocalories per servings
10 minutes	80

Instructions:

1. Preheat the oven to 375°F (190° C). In a bowl, combine honey, olive oil, cinnamon, and a pinch of salt.

2. Toss sliced carrots in the basin until evenly covered. Spread the carrots evenly on a baking sheet lined with parchment paper.

3. Roast the carrots in a warm oven for 20-25 minutes, or until soft and faintly caramelised. Serve hot, and enjoy.

Roasted Zucchini with Herbs

Ingredients:

- 4 medium zucchinis, sliced into rounds
- 2 tablespoons olive oil
- 1 teaspoon dried oregano
- 1 teaspoon dried thyme
- Salt and pepper to taste

Prep time	Kilocalories per servings
15 minutes	100

Instructions:

1. Preheat the oven to 400 °F (200 °C). In a large mixing bowl, combine the zucchini rounds, olive oil, dried oregano, dried thyme, salt and pepper. Spread the seasoned zucchini rounds in a single layer on a parchment-lined or lightly greased baking sheet.
2. Roast in a preheated oven for 15-20 minutes, or until the courgette is soft and gently browned around the edges.
3. Remove from the oven and allow it cool for a few minutes before serving. Enjoy your tasty and healthful roasted zucchini with herbs.

Cucumber and Dill Salad

Ingredients:

- 2 medium cucumbers, thinly sliced
- 1/4 cup fresh dill, chopped
- 1 tablespoon olive oil
- 2 tablespoons apple cider vinegar
- Salt and pepper to taste

Prep time	Kilocalories per servings
10 minutes	50

Instructions:

1. Slice the cucumbers thinly and throw in a mixing dish.
2. Chop the fresh dill and mix it into the bowl with the cucumbers.
3. Drizzle olive oil and apple cider vinegar over the cucumber-dill combination.
4. Season with salt and pepper to taste. Gently toss everything until the cucumbers are uniformly covered.
5. Serve immediately or refrigerate until later. Enjoy this delightful cucumber and dill salad.

Baked Butternut Squash

Ingredients:

- 1 medium-sized butternut squash
- 2 tablespoons olive oil
- Salt and pepper to taste

Prep time	Kilocalories per servings
10 minutes	100

Instructions:

1. Preheat the oven to 400 °F (200 °C). Wash the butternut squash thoroughly, then pat it dry with a clean cloth. Cut the squash in half lengthwise, then scoop out the seeds and stringy pieces with a spoon.

2. Cut each half into 1-inch-thick pieces. Place the squash slices on a baking sheet covered with parchment paper or lightly oiled with olive oil.

3. Drizzle the olive oil over the squash slices and season with salt and pepper as desired. Toss the squash pieces with your hands to coat them evenly in oil and seasoning.

4. Place the slices in a single layer on the baking pan. Bake in the preheated oven for 25-30 minutes, or until the squash is soft and gently browned on the edges.

5. Once baked, remove from the oven and allow to cool slightly before serving.

Steamed Green Beans with Almonds

Ingredients:

- 1 pound fresh green beans, trimmed
- 2 tablespoons slivered almonds
- 1 tablespoon olive oil
- Salt to taste

Prep time	Kilocalories per servings
15 minutes	80

Instructions:

1. Wash the green beans thoroughly with cold water and cut the ends. Put the green beans in a steamer basket over boiling water. Steam for 8-10 minutes, until tender yet still crisp.

2. While the beans are steaming, heat a small skillet on medium heat. Toast

the slivered almonds for 2-3 minutes, until golden brown and fragrant.

3. Keep an eye on them to avoid burning. When the green beans are done, remove them from the steamer and place in a serving dish.

4. Drizzle olive oil over steaming green beans and top with toasted almonds. Season with salt to taste and gently toss to evenly coat the beans. Serve hot as a healthy side dish to your diverticulitis diet.

Quinoa-Stuffed Bell Peppers

Ingredients:

- 4 large bell peppers (any color)
- 1 cup quinoa
- 1 ¾ cups vegetable broth
- 1 can (15 ounces) low-sodium black beans, drained and rinsed
- 1 cup corn kernels (fresh or frozen)
- 1 cup diced tomatoes (canned or fresh)
- 1 teaspoon cumin
- 1 teaspoon chili powder
- Salt and pepper to taste

- Optional toppings: chopped cilantro, avocado slices, shredded cheese (for non-lactose intolerant)

Prep time	Kilocalories per servings
15 minutes	250-300

Instructions:

1. Preheat the oven to 375°F (190° C). Rinse the quinoa with cold water through a fine mesh sieve to remove any bitterness. In a medium saucepan, combine the washed quinoa with the vegetable broth.

2. Bring to a boil, then reduce to a low heat, cover, and simmer for 15-20 minutes, or until the quinoa is cooked and the liquid has been absorbed.

3. While the quinoa is cooking, cut the tops off the bell peppers and remove the seeds and membranes.

4. Put them in a baking dish. In a large mixing bowl, mix together the cooked quinoa, black beans, corn, chopped tomatoes, cumin, paprika, salt and pepper.

5. Mix well. Stuff each bell pepper with the quinoa mixture, gently pressing down to cram it in. Cover the baking dish with foil and bake for 25-30 minutes, until the peppers are cooked.

6. Remove from the oven and allow to cool slightly before serving. Optional toppings include chopped cilantro, avocado slices, and lime wedges.

Mashed Cauliflower

Ingredients:

- 1 large head of cauliflower
- 2 tablespoons olive oil
- 2 cloves garlic, minced
- 1/4 cup low-sodium chicken or vegetable broth
- Salt and pepper to taste

Prep time	Kilocalories per servings
15 minutes	100

Instructions:

1. Rinse the cauliflower thoroughly with cool water. Cut it into florets and discard the stiff stems. Steam the cauliflower florets for 10-12 minutes, or until soft. While the cauliflower is steaming, warm the olive oil in a pan over medium heat. Sauté minced garlic until fragrant, about 1-2 minutes.

2. Once the cauliflower is tender, place it in a food processor or blender. Combine the sautéed garlic, low-sodium broth, salt, and pepper.

3. Blend until smooth and creamy, scraping down the sides of the machine or blender if necessary. Taste and adjust seasoning as needed.

4. Serve mashed cauliflower heated as a healthful and comforting side dish on a diverticulitis diet.

Ingredients:

- 4 cups shredded cabbage (green or red)
- 1 cup shredded carrots
- 1/2 cup Greek yogurt (low-fat or non-fat)
- 2 tablespoons apple cider vinegar
- 1 tablespoon honey
- Salt and pepper to taste

Prep time	Kilocalories per servings
10 minutes	90

Instructions:

1. In a large bowl, combine the shredded cabbage and carrots. In a separate small bowl, mix the Greek yoghurt, apple cider vinegar, honey, salt, and pepper until well blended.

2. Pour the yoghurt mixture over the cabbage and carrots, and toss to coat. Taste and adjust the seasoning as needed.

3. Chill in the refrigerator for at least 30 minutes before serving to enable the flavours to combine.

Day	Breakfast	Lunch	Dinner	Snacks
Monday	Oatmeal with banana slices	Grilled chicken salad	Baked salmon with steamed vegetables	Greek yogurt with honey
Tuesday	Scrambled eggs with spinach	Quinoa and vegetable stir-fry	Turkey meatballs with whole grain pasta	Carrot sticks with hummus
Wednesday	Smoothie (banana, spinach, yogurt)	Lentil soup with whole grain bread	Grilled tilapia with quinoa and steamed broccoli	Apple slices with almond butter
Thursday	Greek yogurt with berries	Grilled vegetable wrap	Chicken and vegetable stir-fry with brown rice	Mixed nuts
Friday	Whole grain toast with avocado	Tuna salad with whole wheat crackers	Baked chicken breast with sweet potato mash	Cottage cheese with pear slices
Saturday	Veggie omelette	Mixed bean salad	Grilled shrimp with quinoa and roasted Brussels sprouts	Trail mix
Sunday	Whole grain pancakes with berries	Turkey and avocado wrap	Vegetable curry with brown rice	Yogurt with granola

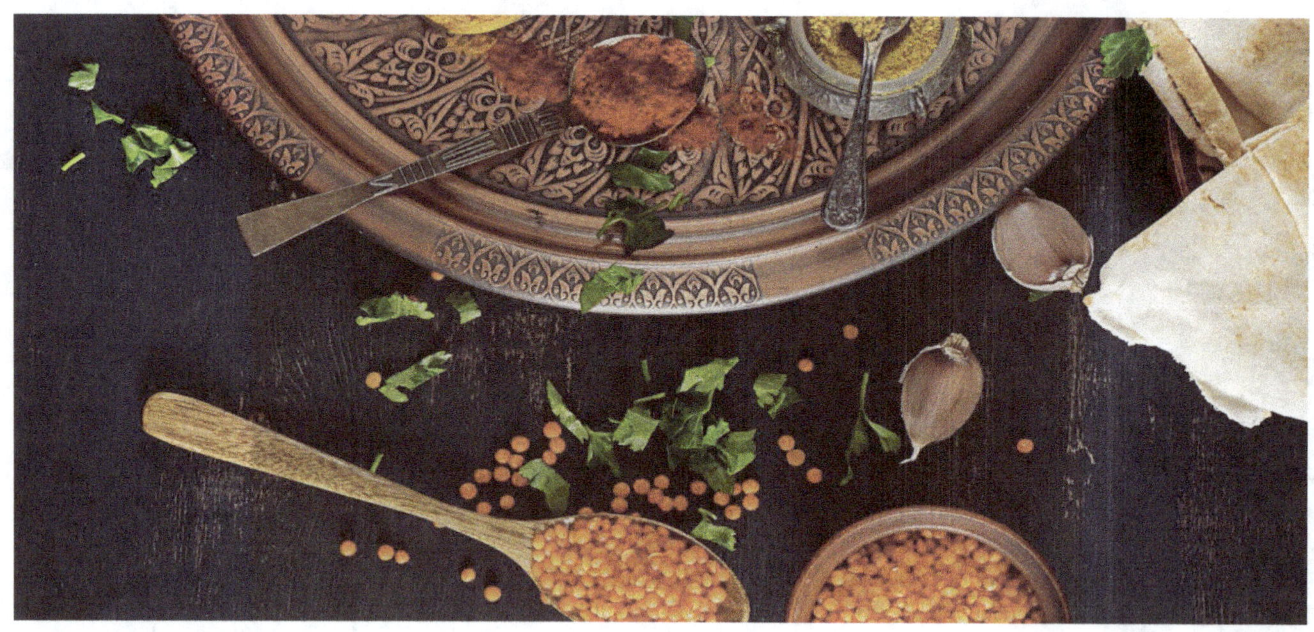

For prevention, consider these suggestions:

1) A balanced diet includes plenty of nutritious grains, fruits, and vegetables.

2) Stay Hydrated: Drink plenty of water to keep things running smoothly.

3) Quit smoking: This can benefit your overall gut health.

4) Maintain a Healthy Weight: Regular exercise and a well-balanced diet will help you stay in shape and lower your risk of flare-ups.

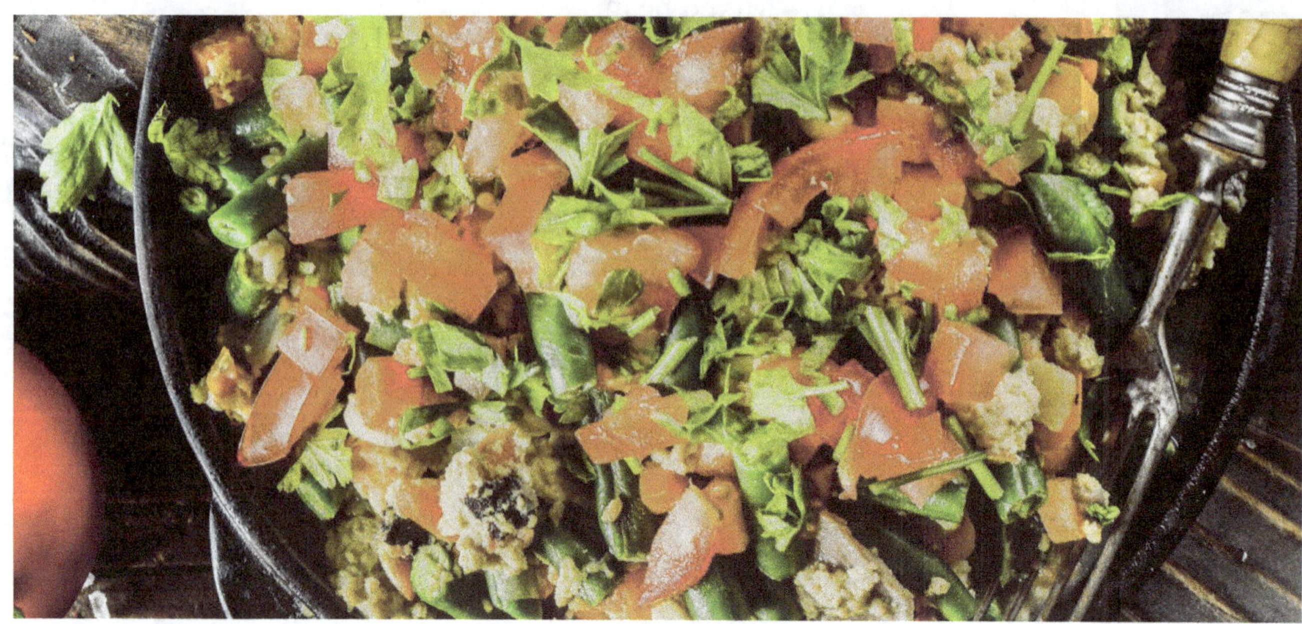

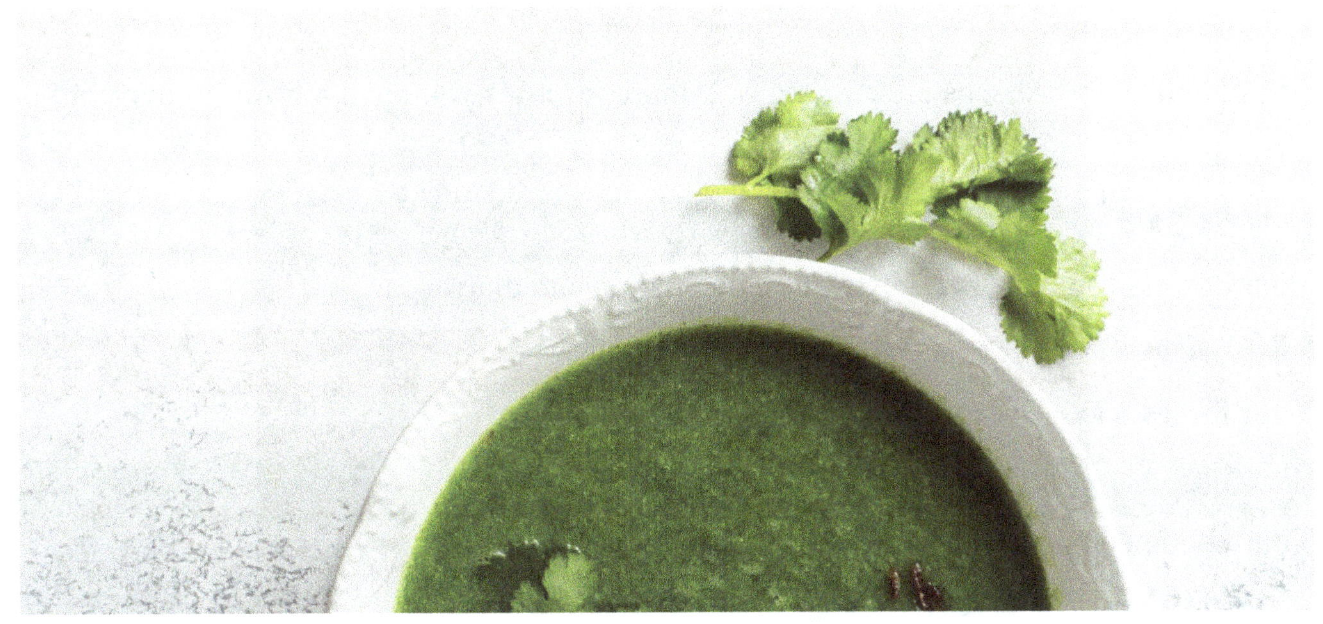

Importance of Diet in Managing Symptoms

The Diverticulitis Drama unfolds. Diverticulosis occurs when small pouches, or diverticula, grow in the walls of the large intestine.

Consider these pouches to be small nooks where trouble can brew. But there's a narrative twist: when these pouches get inflamed, it causes diverticulitis.

Consider this:

Your immune system, which is always on alert, senses a problem. It mobilises, boosts blood flow, and transports disease-fighting cells to the scene. What was the result? Inflammation. Suddenly, those once-innocent diverticula have become the focus of attention.

The Mysterious Symptoms

Tummy troubles: The most common symptom is pain in the lower left side of your abdomen, though some people may have discomfort on the right side as well.

Mealtime Drama:

The pain usually worsens after eating but improves after you have a bowel movement or release gas.

Constipation versus Diarrhoea:

Your bowels could alternate between constipation and diarrhoea.

Bloody Business:

Your faeces may occasionally contain blood.

Bloating:

Your abdomen may inflate and feel like a balloon.

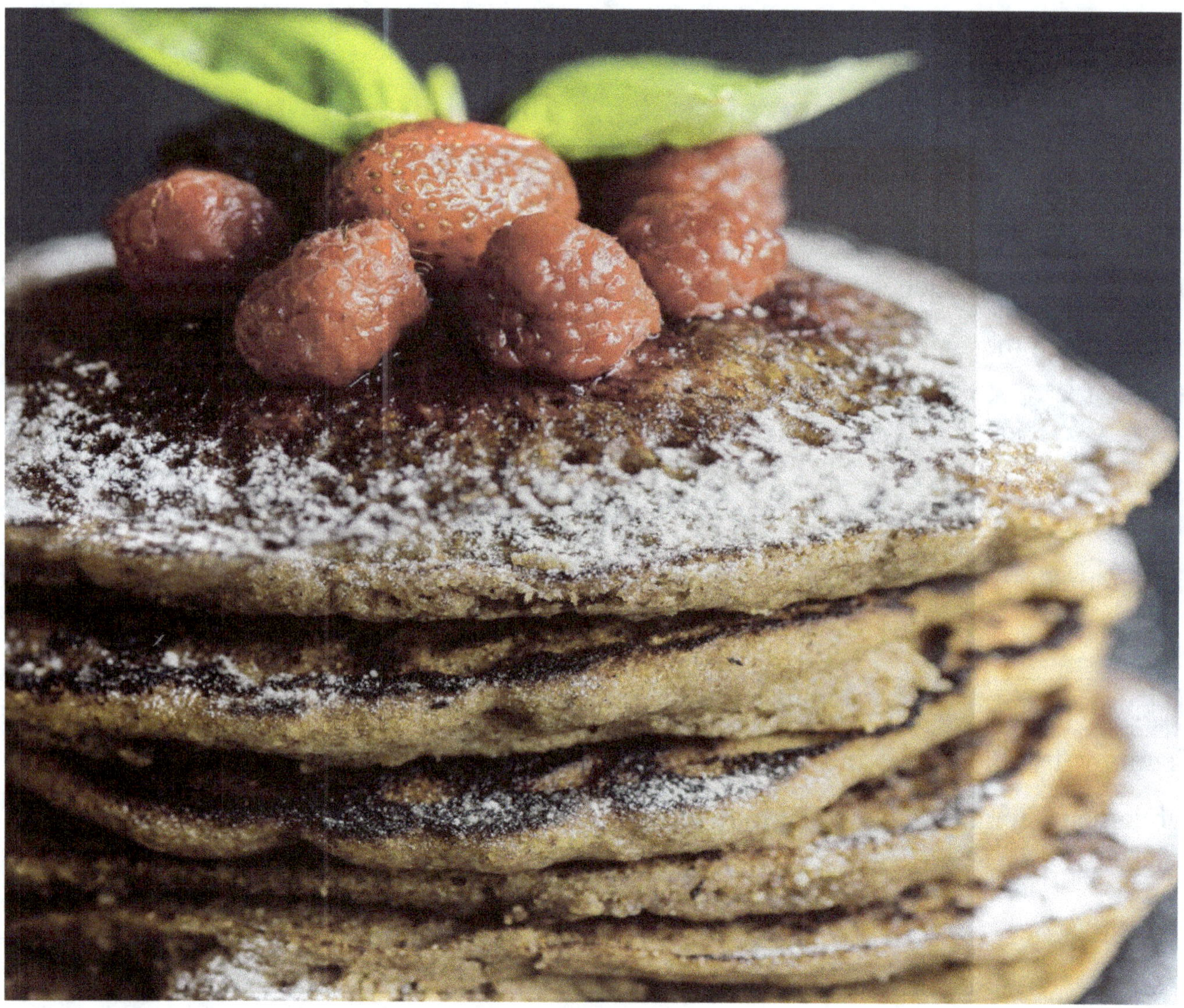